TIME
and
TIDES

*One Man's Battle for Survival
Through the Eyes of His Wife*

VINALIES INTERNATIONALES GOLD MEDAL RECIPIENT

J. MAKI

Copyright © 2023 J. Maki

All rights reserved.

This book, or parts thereof, may not be reproduced in any form or by any means without written permission from the author, except for brief passages for purposes of reviews. For more information, contact the publisher at support@publishandgo.com.

ISBN 978-1-961093-00-3 (Hardcover Book)
ISBN 978-1-961093-01-0 (Softcover Book)
ISBN 978-1-961093-02-7 (eBook)

Published by Silversmith Press–Houston, Texas
www.silversmithpress.com

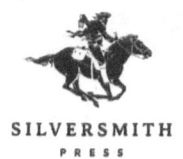

Contents

About the Book 4

Dedication 5

In Appreciation 6

Preface 7

Day One, Of the Rest of My Life 11

The First 90 Days 16

Day By Day 37

Week 5 41

Surgery 45

Hospice 216

Afterword 309

About the Book

This is the jaw-dropping, two-year odyssey of a wife trying to save her husband from a stage four cancer diagnosis.

JAMES MORRISON HALDY

Dedication

This book is dedicated to caregivers and their patients everywhere, especially my husband and cancer patient, Fred Maki.

In Appreciation

―・•●•・―

Special appreciation needs to be given to many who cared for Fred and me.

First is to my Mom and Dad, whose genes I am, whose spirits I have, whose strength I draw my strength from, and whose spirits walk with me daily.

We can never give enough thanks to the wonderful people at the Fox Chase Cancer Center. God bless you, one and all, every day. Your warmth, your smiles, your kindness, your caring, your support, your consideration, and your professionalism helped us endure an unbearable situation.

And especially to Fred's team of doctors.

Preface

It's Not Your Story

It's been suggested that I begin from the beginning of this journey. Day One of the rest of my life, as I think of it. But in case you only read the beginning, I want you to remember one thing that has stayed with me throughout—something I was glad to learn in the early weeks and something I was reminded about many times: The story is not mine to tell.

In the first few weeks after we were diagnosed, I wanted to scream day and night. With everyone I saw—toll takers, grocery check-out clerks, the person standing next to me—I could barely hear what they were saying, and I wanted to yell at everyone that my husband had cancer! And not the kind where you just cut it out, but the kind that kills. The urge was constant and overwhelming.

Truthfully, we were deeply in shock, barely able to

speak. As the first hours and days wore on, my survival instincts kicked in, and I went into action. Getting to the right doctor was paramount. My personality type is to move quickly to action, and along with that comes the need for communication. So, after things were set in motion, I felt the need to start telling our friends. As I inquired about whom my husband wanted to tell, the answer was no one. No one included his parents!

I would have pushed the issue in our normal life, but this situation was not normal. Things are important for a few moments, then the rush of the waterfall overwhelms you repeatedly, and each time you surface briefly for air, less and less appears to be important. Surviving the moment takes all your energy.

After a few weeks, I was lamenting to my mother that my husband could not tell his parents or daughter. I thought I would have to call them, for surely they needed to know. My mother, who teaches nursing, had been gathering information from her contacts for me. She simply said, "It's his story to tell."

As soon as she said those words, I knew it was true. As maddening as it was, this was my husband's story to tell or not to tell—his way, his time.

My role was to support, care for and love him, be strong for him, communicate, stand by, help in any way, be patient, listen, be his advocate, and be hopeful. I am the caregiver, but it's his story.

Cancer, An Epidemic

In 2003, it is expected that we in the US will have 1.2 million new cases of cancer diagnosed. There are over 300 types of cancer. Over 550,000 people will die this year from cancer. Esophageal and stomach cancers are not the leading types of cancer. But they are some of the worst—for treatment and survivability. Cancer is the second-leading cause of death in the US after heart disease. These and many other statistics are available on the American Cancer Society website.

After one year, we have learned the awful truth about Fred's cancer: 80% of all esophageal cancer patients die within five years.

Esophageal cancer is a very deadly enemy. It spreads to new locations and sets up shop in advanced cases. It changes itself to become more resistant to treatment.

When it moves to a new location, it grabs healthy cells to surround it and changes those cells, making them resistant to treatment. These cells are the "feeder" cells and protect the cancer cells. They are very effective.

Day One, Of the Rest of My Life

—–·•·—–

The image is permanently imprinted in my mind of the look on the doctor's face—the first person who knew the awful truth. He was ashen, obviously upset about something, and avoiding eye contact. I knew instantly that this was not going to be good news. But we just weren't prepared; it wasn't supposed to happen to us. He was so young.

Day One was five days earlier when I picked up a cell phone message from my husband. I was out for my day's schedule, trying to find business in a market that was spiraling downward. His message said, "Well, I just got a strange call from the doctor's office to go immediately to the emergency room and get blood, so I'll see you later." All of my alarms went off. We knew he hadn't been feeling well for some time—low energy, quick exhaustion with minimal physical exertion. He kept saying he was just out of shape.

There were other symptoms, as I would learn later.

I called our General Physician, who had referred him to a Digestive Disease Specialist when they got back the recent blood results, and finally followed my husband's trail to the emergency room of our regional hospital. His hemoglobin was 6, and a normal male's level was 16. It was so low that he could have just dropped dead while walking around. A specialist was going to see him in the ER while he was getting three units of blood. We were impressed with the efficiency and care taken with the blood typing. It was all fascinating, the "keys" to matching the patient to his units of blood. He was cold and got a little colder during the transfusion. We weren't thinking, "Why does he need blood?" We were relieved to be at the hospital and for him to receive the precious serum of life, expecting he would instantly feel great and we'd be on our merry way.

The specialist arrived, and I dutifully asked him where he went to school. He brightened up and spoke of his internship down south, proud of the well-known doctors he had worked with. He and his resident probed, took a stool sample, checked his vital signs, and asked about his symptoms and history. It was then that I learned that he had trouble swallowing. "For how long?" asked the specialist. "About a year," answered my husband.

The specialist's eyes glanced at me and recognized my look of disbelief. "A year?" I said, dumbfounded. More probing; no pain anywhere. "Any family history of cancer?" he asked casually. Personal information is rarely shared within the family—Finns are notoriously private. We said we'd check, but the doctor didn't seem to think it was important.

Later that night, we walked outside into a beautiful, late-summer evening. Fred was looking rosier due to the transfusion. We had no information about why he needed blood, or so it seemed at the time. We stopped for a video on the way home. Our animals reminded us that we were gone entirely too long. The next day we received a call with some scheduled diagnostic tests, none of which sounded very intrusive. We settled into our regular routine, barely thinking of the cause of the bleeding and never suspected a life-threatening reason.

Tuesday arrived, and we went to the specialist's

office for an endoscopy. A lot of effort was made to educate us on the procedure and the aftercare. I was the designated driver and would wait for the procedure and recovery for 1-2 hours. I left to run an errand to the bookstore nearby, leaving my cell phone number in case he was finished before I returned. I had been in the bookstore for five minutes when they called. I was surprised that he finished so quickly and took that as a good sign. They ushered me into the recovery area, where my husband was sipping soda. Our lighthearted conversation stopped when I saw the doctor's face. He was ashen, obviously upset about something, and avoided eye contact when I said, "You don't look well." He paused and then said, "It's not good." I said, "What do you mean?" And he handed me a picture, saying, "This is the picture of Fred's esophagus." I was a biology and pre-med major in college. I know what healthy cells should look like, and I knew these were not healthy cells. These were a bulbous ulcerated mass. Shock waves ripped through me. My husband was not coherent enough to understand. "So now what?" I asked. "What are the options?" He said he took a biopsy, and we would need those results first—they would tell if it was malignant. And there was more. He nearly choked when he said he couldn't scope very far because there was a tumor the size of his fist. He was holding his fist in front of my face, and his eyes looked pleadingly at me, as if to ask me to relieve him of speaking about this. At that point, my husband said, "What's the matter?" I covered him with my upper body to shield him from more harm. The tears were streaking down my face. He said again. "What's wrong?" I said, "It's good that you are big, strong, and tough because you're going to need to be."

In hindsight, I'm surprised I said this because my mind was working on multiple thought paths. The doctor never said the C word; he only called it an ulcerous tumor.

From high school biology, I remember: *"Cancer is a sudden, uncontrolled cellular growth."*

The First 90 Days

Thursday, September 12, 2002

Reading Hospital Emergency Room, Hemoglobin levels: 6.7, getting two units of blood; type A positive. Dizzy, shortness of breath, gray in color, difficulty with food going down into the stomach, some vomiting, weight loss that has been intentional, no energy.

Friday–Monday, September 13–16, 2002

Going on with our days, but something has changed. It's not urgent, but now we'll know why Fred hasn't been feeling well for months. We don't talk about it.

Tuesday, September 17, 2002

The first endoscopy was very quick, and the picture was of gross, bulbous, ulcerous, bloody esophagus and upper stomach walls. Not good. A biopsy revealed that it is most likely cancer.

Shock! My world stopped; it can't be...What can be done? Poor Fred, why me? Why Fred? What would my world be like in the future? Stop this! Fred will live; he will beat this. I must have more info.

Time and motion don't exist.

No feelings.

Should be fear.

Shock, disbelief, must be a mistake.

No thoughts, must think, can't think.

Wednesday, September 18, 2002

I meet Cindy, a pastor at the YMCA, and ask her to pray for Fred. I break down. She says she has a parishioner, Kurt, who has something similar and found the best doctor in the country right here in Philadelphia. She will get me his name.

Cindy calls with the parishioner's name and telephone number. I talk to Kurt, and he tells me there's hope. He's waiting for surgery, and things look good. Initially, they don't give good odds, but as treatment progresses, they get better. Dr. Goldberg is the best in the country. Kurt's surgery is next week.

Thursday, September 19, 2002

"The CT Scan results are better than expected," says the local doctor. There is no liver or lung involvement, possibly some lymph nodes. The cancer is only in the esophagus and stomach. This is supposed to be good news. We request a referral to Dr. Goldberg at Fox Chase Cancer Center. I can't believe I'm doing this.

Devastation.
Is there a future for us?
How will we live?
Nothing is the same.
Nothing is.
All seems destroyed.
The sounds are gone.

There are no voices, no music.

Friday, September 20, 2002

Harvest continues. Fred tells Ike, our friend and fellow viticulturist. It's his first telling.

Saturday, September 21, 2002

Fred is sick, has diarrhea, and is unable to eat. They said he might need another transfusion. It's the weekend. I call the doctor's office. I'm not sure if I should be alarmed. No one calls back. We're alone. My mother is on call 24 hours a day, 7 days a week.

Sunday, September 22, 2002

We disgorge champagne together—the slow, tedious, manual last steps in the multi-year champagne-making process. I wonder if this is our last time. Not knowing a prognosis is terrible. Fred is destroyed emotionally. I checked the Fox Chase website. The treatment is done by a three-person team: the surgeon, the oncologist, and the radiologist.

Monday, September 23, 2002

I call Dr. Goldberg's office. We can't waste time. We need to see the other physician ASAP. His assistant, Rose, hears me and, within an hour, calls back with the other appointments. I also asked the local hospital for a referral to their team. Kurt said he had the chemotherapy and radiation at the local hospital, coordinated with Fox Chase. Fox Chase is over an hour's drive each way. It's good to get a second opinion.

Tuesday, September 24, 2002

Waiting, not knowing if there is hope, not believing there isn't, but praying there is. Fred is decimated.

Wednesday, September 25, 2002

Fred asks for Kurt's number. I'm shocked when he calls, talks to the son, and asks how Kurt is. The surgery was a success.

Thursday, September 26, 2002

AM: At the doctor's office in Reading, he spends 15 minutes talking about why he doesn't have a nicer office, lots of gross descriptions of cancer treatment, offering little hope, and the latest information. He orders three units of blood and suggests it is time to call in all favors. We all have to die sometime! He gives Fred a prescription for a large dose of Zoloft. We leave with more shock.

PM: Fox Chase Cancer Center is a nice friendly facility. We meet Dr. Goldberg, 60-ish, bow tie, not wordy. He reviews the tests and says we need all the treatments—chemotherapy, radiation, and surgery—to give Fred a chance. In the end, he said he thought he could help. That was the first time we heard that. But it didn't lift the gloom. Hope was still elusive. I must mobilize Fred's fight. All night I spent killing the cancer cells.

Friday, September 27, 2002

We travel back to Fox Chase for an appointment with Dr. Cheng, the medical oncologist. Anne Peligrino, Dr. Cheng's nurse, meets with us. She tells us several times to call her with any questions. I guess she's observing Fred. Finally, Dr. Cheng arrives. He's friendlier, more personable, and more talkative than Dr. Goldberg. He says Fred's cancer is big and advanced. He talks about a new drug trial. Fred is big and strong; they will give him as much as possible without hurting him. He talks about chemotherapy drugs and the cycle. They want to do their own tests, and then the surgeon will decide the course of treatment. The traditional approach is surgery then chemotherapy and radiation. Their experience shows that the results are better if chemotherapy and radiation are performed first. He suggests that they may be able to stop the bleeding, at least partially. He asks if we can stay and says he will talk to another doctor to complete a procedure as soon as possible. It's an endoscopy. We say he just had one. They say their specialists know how to do things specific to cancer treatment. Ok. He gives Fred prescriptions for sleeping pills (Ambien) and Ativan for anxiety.

We are waiting to see the radiologist, Dr. Konski. His nurse, Eileen, meets with us. Everyone gives us lots of reading material and their business cards. They tell us to call anytime.

Later, Dr. Haulouska meets with us, and they immediately take Fred. I wait in a small waiting area with a TV. Anne stops by to sit with me. Everyone smiles and is friendly. Dr. H. tells me he stopped much of the bleeding, took biopsies, and enlarged the junction between the stomach and the esophagus where the big tumor is. This should help Fred with eating. The only problem was that he couldn't reach the area between his stomach and pancreas for a biopsy. We're amazed that they were able to mobilize to do this procedure on the spot. We leave with a schedule of tests for the next week. Fred is relaxed from the anesthesia.

Saturday, September 28, 2002

Fred can eat better. We're glad to have found Fox Chase. The harvest continues. It's a good thing we have two workers this year.

Sunday, September 29, 2002

Fred is in a panic. He is very agitated and begging for help. I call the Fox Chase emergency number and get to a nurse supervisor. She is calming and talks us through what is going on. She says it is good that Fred is aware of his emotional pain; it is part of the natural grieving process. He is going to lose a part of himself. This is one of the phases. What are the phases? This does not comfort Fred. Later, he describes how his body is racing 100 miles an hour inside. We determine that maybe it's the Zoloft and don't take any more.

Monday through Sunday, September 30–October 6, 2002

Monday: he is calmer without the Zoloft.

We're waiting for news about when Fred will start treatment. We visit Fox Chase daily for pre-surgery, port surgery, tests, and radiation setup. There's no problem with the CT scan. His radiation setup requires mold-making, and Fred has difficulty holding his arms over his head. Finally, they get this done. Then he gets a tattoo to mark the spot for radiation. Next, a special MRI is used to set up his position for radiation. He can't keep his arms still. We are there for hours. They give him Ativan under the tongue. It possibly helps. The technician works with Fred to give him breaks. He barely makes it through the test.

I talk to Anne about the treatment schedule. There's nothing yet. She comes down to sit with me while I wait for the tests. I keep asking questions and rephrasing questions. I'm looking for a prognosis. They don't take patients they can't help. They won't give false hope.

We're getting more comfortable going to Fox Chase. Everyone there has cancer; we're all in the same boat. There is always someone in a worse situation. Fred is very quiet.

Bonnie, our neighbor, is in frequent contact. She does charity work for the Look Good, Feel Good Program to help cancer patients. She brings up food and offers assistance. She helps check in on the pets when we're at the hospital.

Friday: Fred is going crazy and saying he needs help. I call Anne and get a referral for a psychiatrist. She says they have the test results so far—nothing new—but Fred can't be part of the new drug trial because of the spot outside his stomach. Finally, I realize that this could be another cancer. What more is there? I don't tell Fred.

All weekend he is a basket case, unable to move or talk. He doesn't want to hear me talk on the phone; I usually cry.

He asks about the treatment, and I tell him he can't be in the trial. We discuss this several times and prepare questions for Monday. He asks, "What if that new drug is the one that would really help me? What do I have to lose?"

Monday through Friday, October 7–11, 2002

Monday: Anne tells me what the schedule is. I ask about the new drug. She says she'll have Dr. Cheng call me. He calls later and explains further why Fred couldn't participate in the trial. I ask, "What if that is the drug that would really help?" And he says, "It's possible. There's no conclusion yet. After the PET scan, the doctors will have a conference later this week and decide on a course of action. We plan on chemotherapy and radiation next week."

Wednesday: he has a PET scan. This gives very fine detail and shows any additional cancer. They say the test costs as much as a car. Before that, he takes an Ativan. We talk to the technician about the problem with holding his arms during tests. The technician is more schedule-oriented. Fred comes out, holding his arm in visible pain. His body is shaking from being in one position. I try to be sympathetic. I give him his lunch. We have to rush to a meeting with the psychiatrist, Dr. Z. I go ahead and get the car, so he has time to recover.

Fred says he wants his emotional self back. Dr. Z. says that's a good start and prescribes Remeron for depression and talks about using the drugs for the best help. I think that Fred should talk about his feelings. He only wants to get drugs. I remember—it's not my story.

Saturday, October 12, Champagne Day 2002

Finally, the day arrives. I do my best to prepare. This year we have an international guest—Uncle Jack from Germany—and three aunts from Ohio. They all arrive with my mother on Friday. I meet them at the Coventry Tea Room, but I can't eat. They all know about Fred, but no one speaks about it.

On Saturday, Fred is able to participate. No one notices that he holds on to the counter and leans on me.

Most of our work crew doesn't know. It's the only way I can survive now—by pretending everything is the same. I feel like I'm in the twilight zone.

Sunday, October 13, 2002

We wait for Monday when the killing of the alien begins.

Monday through Monday, October 14–21, 2002, Treatment Week 1.

Confusion at the blood lab. We're a late addition to the schedule, and they have to work us in. Dr. Cheng comes to see us and finalize the papers. He has ordered the new drug. He gives us a prescription for anti-nausea. We wait. I have a moment of horror at what's happening to us. People look away as tears stream down my face. I don't think Fred sees my tears. He's living in his own horror.

We enter the infusion room; it is a big area with multiple open stations, not separate rooms. Fred was here two weeks ago for a transfusion. The nurse talks to us about everything, encourages our questions, and says, "Always ask or call right away; don't wait till your next visit." They give me lots of reading material. Some are duplicates. They are very good at communication. They start the pre-medications: Benedryl 25 mg IV, Decadron 10 mg IV, Tagomet 300 mg IV, Kytril 1 mg IV, and saline. Then we start with Cisplatin (55 mg IV) and post-hydration with 1000 cc of saline, followed by Paclitaxel (110 mg IV) and more saline. I sit with Fred. He asks me to be quiet, as others have it tough, many tougher than he. When the first chemotherapy drug is started, we make an imaginary toast to show that the killing of the alien has begun. I bring lunch for Fred. He doesn't like to see me eating. At home, I eat in the kitchen. After the infusion is well underway, I go to the cafeteria. It's spacious and full of daylight. The walk outside is pleasant. There is an open, friendly feeling everywhere. Finally, the infusion is complete, and they connect a "fanny pack" to a CADD pump that delivers 440 mg/day of 5-fluorouracil (5-FU) 24 hours a day, seven days a week, Monday through Friday.

At 5:30 p.m., we leave the infusion room with the

fanny pack for the third drug, 5-FU. Then we go to radiation. We wait because we are not on the schedule yet. By 6:30 p.m., we leave. Bonnie will have dinner in the oven for us when we get home.

Tuesday, October 22, 2002

Radiation is scheduled for 7:00 a.m. It takes only 10 minutes.

The infusion fanny pack makes a noise like the alien's "member" in the Alien movie. We laugh a little.

Wednesday, October 23, 2002

We go to Harrisburg in the morning to present our marketing idea to the PA Wineries Association Board. He is wearing his fanny pack of chemotherapy drugs. It makes a whirring sound occasionally. He dresses to hide it. The meeting goes well; no one seems to notice. They want us to prepare the idea for a vote at next year's annual meeting. I say we don't have time; we need to start now. Fred is happy that I am working on this with him. We plan our next steps. I think this could be a good project for Fred for the winter.

Later, I talk to Kurt, the other patient. He's very sore from surgery and has leg pain. He was hospitalized for only ten days—something about an infection. We can't attend the support group with him on Monday; Fred is in the infusion room all day. Kurt doesn't think they can go either; he's returning to Fox Chase on Thursday about the leg and hip pain.

Thursday, October 24, 2002

Fred is getting nauseous. Anne prescribes a stronger drug.

Friday – Sunday, October 25-27, 2002

Fred is nauseous every day, more or less. I see his infusion nurse at the hospital. She recommends some foods: "Try popsicles; they are easy on the throat. He needs more liquids to clean out the chemotherapy drugs from his kidneys. Drink sodas, anything, but drink!"

Sunday night: Cindy leaves a message saying that

Kurt has died! She didn't want Fred to see this in the paper. Kurt is the person whose path we are following. I am panicked. Mom says it's probably due to complications. I will call Cindy on Monday. I will keep this from Fred.

Monday, October 28, 2002

Infusion room day: I was able to schedule us for bloodwork at 7:30 a.m. I go swimming and get back when he gets into the infusion room. I ask about infections. We're getting more familiar with the hospital. They have a unique culture. I walk around to see more of the facility.

Tuesday, October 29, 2002

Radiation only: Fred is still nauseous. At night, he decides he wants to get together with our wine group for dinner. He's afraid he may not be able to in the future. Bonnie tries to make the arrangements. One couple seems unresponsive. Fred is upset and only focused on this. He wants to know that the dinner has been set up. I try to be diplomatic; we are working on it. He says he's going down to Bonnie's. I follow him. This is the first time he's going anywhere but Fox Chase. They are surprised, and he wants to know, "What's the problem?" He doesn't understand why everyone doesn't make themselves available. He would do so for them. He is in a hurry. It may be the last time we gather. He cries.

Wednesday, October 30, 2002

Fred is getting more nauseous. He can hardly eat and feels sick. He doesn't talk.

Thursday, October 31, 2002

This night we are meeting with our wine-tasting group for dinner. He gets dressed but is silent. He asks about his hair. We meet everyone, and after 20 minutes, he is so sick that we go home. I go back to have dinner. I cry constantly and tell his story. I eat with tears streaming down my face. Everyone is silent. I tell them about Kurt and that I am more scared now and worried about infection. I say, "Fred is tough and strong, and that is helping him get through this."

They say, "Yes, Fred is tough," and "He looks good," not like they expected. I leave so they can enjoy some of their dinner.

Friday, November 1, 2002

I call Anne. He is still nauseous, more so, and can't eat. We say he is OK on Mondays. Is that the steroid?

The weekend goes quietly. The red wine fermentations are slow.

Saturday, November 2, 2002

We go to Cape May for the day with Tashie, our dog. We drive the slow way through southern NJ. It's a very busy and beautiful day in Cape May; I'm surprised at the number of year-round residents. We go to the Lobster Pot Restaurant, which is located on a large wharf, and Fred orders oysters on the half-shell. He says his eating is much easier. They have a huge fish market. We drink beer and sit on the dock. As I drive home, he gets agitated, so I go faster. The road is one lane in each direction, and I get stuck behind a truck for 15 miles. He practically starts screaming and thrashing in the car. I don't know why he's so agitated. Finally, I pull over. He doesn't talk for the rest of the ride home.

Monday, November 4, 2002, Week 2

The infusion room: Donna and Marie come to visit. Fred says, "Okay." They bring flowers and stuff and come to the infusion room. Fred is animated and tells them about his experience. It feels like it was good for him. The nurse confirms that we can get Fred steroids to help with nausea. I get the prescription filled at the pharmacy near the hospital. Fred doesn't want our local pharmacy to know. He always eats well on Mondays and has energy. He's a bit of a bear, too.

Tuesday, November 5, 2002

He is starting steroids, with radiation, every day. We see Dr. Z. Fred talks mostly about the drugs. He asks again about his hair. There are no signs of change yet. On the way home, he points out the cemeteries on the ride to and from the hospital. He says he can't stand to look. They were everywhere on the ride back from Cape May—that's probably why he was upset. We put our hands to the sides of our faces to blind us from seeing the cemeteries on the way home.

Wednesday through Friday, November 6–8, 2002

Things smooth out. He can eat and is a little pumped up. He becomes more awake and active. He wants to eat everything.

Day By Day

People say, "I don't know how you do it." I respond that I go day by day and that I cry a lot. I also talk to myself. I only think about what needs to be done today and don't worry about everything else. My priorities are food and shelter.

Sleep escapes me as I look hard in the dark for life,

I listen intently for sounds of his breathing.

Terror in the morning with the first hints of day,

I check hesitantly for his chest heaving.

The pain of living in hope for a future.

We ask and ask a different way,

Looking for encouragement

We will be cured.

The pain of knowing there may not be a future.

Saturday, November 9, 2002

We go to Gettysburg, and he is very weak. We drive ourselves to the self-guided tour stops. We have both read "Killer Angels" about the Battle of Gettysburg. This is a somber place, and for a little while, we forget our hell.

Monday, November 10, 2002, Week 4

Things seem more routine. Mom comes to visit in the infusion room. My excursions from the infusion room are getting longer. I pretend that this is our new life and that things are normalizing.

Fred is eating well but needs to drink more liquids to flush out his kidneys. He is getting hyperactive, wants everything done now, and starts buying things. Finally, we start pressing the red wines. Late this year, they may be very good.

Tuesday through Thursday, November 11–13, 2002

Fred drives himself and leaves at 6:00 a.m. I get a break. I ask Dad to visit Fred. I am crying when I say that Fred can't tell his own dad, and it would be nice if he could come.

Saturday, November 14, 2002

We're at Valley Forge National Park, Visitor's center, a movie about the winter encampment, and a tour with a ranger. We walk in a group. The sun is out, and it's 75 degrees. I walk close to Fred, link arms, and match his pace. He is slow; he's getting weak but tries not to show it. When the ranger pauses, Fred sits or lies on the grass. I notice a few people looking at him. I also look to see what they see. He gets tired, and we decide to go home.

Sunday, November 15, 2002

Fred asks that if I knew something about his chances, would I tell him? And he also asks if I'm keeping anything from him; I say, "No, I'm not," and I'm unsure if I am.

Our phone is mercilessly silent. Everyone is surprised at Fred's appearance; he still has hair—that is the first thing people ask about. There is an image of how cancer patients look. If you don't look anemic and half-dead, they don't think it's bad. It feels like they want to dismiss the devastation and go back to the way things were. So do we.

Week 5

Dad comes to the infusion room to visit. Fred talks about his experience. We have a nice visit over lunch. Fred calls his daughter when we get home. That is a big deal.

We're waiting for the treatment to finish. There's no trip to Cape Cod this Thanksgiving.

I drive to Reading every day to pick up two workers. I work with them in the vineyard. We are pre-pruning, and we're doing extra this year, cutting out all the old wood. I determine that we must do this now; it's our only chance to make it in the spring. The vines don't wait. My determined self takes over; I pick them up at 7:00 a.m., work ahead of them to mark the vines for cutting, get lunch, and drive them back, then I do my own work every day. I hope my back holds out.

December, After Chemotherapy and Radiation

Fred gives me a picture and says if he doesn't make it, that's the picture he wants to be published. It's a picture of him and me on one of our mountain climbing trips.

We live in a vacuum without sound, color, or feeling. We don't talk about the cancer. We talk about the new wine organization and how important it is for us. It will change the future.

We are devastated, he physically, and both of us mentally and emotionally.

There is no floor

Only a barren black-and-white landscape

No sun, no moon

Time has stopped

Only the seasons continue

As we stand still.

We are in a time warp; the usual holiday sensations are absent, good and bad.

I continue to do our work for the vineyard and the winery; I have no time and cannot try to get consulting work for myself. The economy is very bad. Next year will be better. Fred gets anxious periodically about our new winery marketing organization, but nothing is happening. I start a flurry of activity. He wants this to happen. I will make this happen for him.

We see the surgeon. He explains the details of the surgery. We set the date for January 7. Diagnostic tests follow. We know the tumor has shrunk a lot, and the spot outside his stomach is resolved. Relief! There is a chance he may keep some of his stomach. We are afraid to hope.

One day, Fred goes to the FedEx regional center to ship our entry to this year's Vinalies International Wine Competition in Paris, France. It was a big effort to discover how to send it. $300 per entry, six bottles, and about $300 to ship! He is quiet when he comes home and tired. He tells me two days later that he was embarrassed because his hands shook so badly that he couldn't complete the form. He had to ask the clerk to fill it out for him and explain that he has an illness. I tell him that I'm sorry that he had a bad time. Sometime during chemotherapy and radiation, this shaking started; I can't remember when I first noticed it. I guess it will go away.

Fred grows more anxious as the month continues. I remember that Cindy had said that our time together is sacred no matter what happens. It's true.

Meanwhile, the Patient is...

Fighting the war,

Afraid to face the light of day,

Reeling with disbelief and shocked beyond belief,

Terrified of the dark and of what comes next,

Steeling himself for the fight,

Unable to move, think, care,

Alone beyond connection,

Viewing from a lonely island

That he alone knows.

Surgery

As the day approaches, the fear mounts. We get quieter and quieter. There were no incoming phone calls. Thank you. We know how big the surgery is, how complex, and that some don't survive. I am catatonic. It takes all of my strength to get through the day. We meet with Zubie (our nickname), the psychiatrist. He listens to Fred describe the past days' events. Then he says, "Of course you are worried. We, the doctors, talk about this in medical terms that sound scary. But the surgery is performed every day. Once you're on the other side, you'll be recovering just like from any surgery."

We adjust; this must be the next phase—waiting until you're on the other side.

The final check—nurse talks to us very slowly as we wait for the surgeon. They check everything four times: "Name, address, do you know what you are here for?" He tells us that after the surgery and the recovery, Fred will no longer be able to smoke or drink. We look at each other, and I say, "We don't smoke, and we make wine. Are you saying he can't drink wine?" The nurse says, "That's right." I say, "Are you sure?" We have repeatedly asked every doctor since Fred was diagnosed. The nurse pauses and says that's what they tell all patients, but he will ask Dr. G. The nurse leaves, and I say to Fred, "Don't worry; if we have to change our lives, we'll sell the winery and move somewhere else." (I can't believe someone wouldn't have told us this!)

I kiss Fred in the prep room before surgery and say, "I'll see you in ICU—on the other side."

See You On The Other Side

We should have danced more,

We should have laughed more,

We should have loved more every day.

We should have kissed more, touched more, and cared more,

Every day.

Meet me on the other side,

Please be on the other side

And we will dance more, laugh more, and love more every day.

We will kiss more, touch more, and care more every day.

Two minutes after they take Fred to surgery, the nurse returns to say he checked with Dr. G., and wine differs from alcohol; wine is fine. Yes, of course, he can have wine. Mom waits with me; we have lunch in the cafeteria. She sees a nurse whom she taught some time ago and who is now head of nursing at Fox Chase. It's a 7-hour surgery. Suddenly, Dr. Goldberg is there; I can't read anything on his face. We sit away from the lounge, and he says Fred is fine; the surgery went well. Relief pours from me. He is excited. The chemotherapy and radiation worked extremely well. The tumor and areas of the esophagus were "Like a concrete mass." He was able to save over half of his stomach! Fred will be so happy! I can see him in about an hour in ICU.

He's overjoyed to be alive and to learn that a large

portion of his stomach is still intact. We had been afraid to talk about this after the initial shock of knowing he might not have any stomach. His first question, though, is, "What about wine?" Food and wine are big parts of our life. We couldn't fathom life without it.

He has tubes everywhere—seven tubes, two in the nose, two large chest tubes for drainage, IVs for medications and liquids, and a catheter. I sit while he awakens for a time. Twenty-four hours later, he's out of the ICU and in a patient room. There's lots of care.

Day 2: The body is making sounds—good sounds. They get him up and walking. He needs a staff to untangle the tubes.

Day 3: He goes into a-fibrillation. I am looking at him while his monitor goes erratic. Half an hour goes by; his pulse is 190. They do an EKG, give him a shot, no change, the cardiologist arrives within thirty minutes (this happens to 30% of the patients with major chest surgery), and they whisk him back to the ICU. I cry again as I drive home, just when I thought the worst was over... I am good at crying in the car now. I think I must be at the bottom. I couldn't possibly have any more emotions. Later that night, he stabilizes. He's given another drug, Amiodarone.

The weekend in the ICU: He can't drink or eat. He has to sit up; it's too uncomfortable to lie flat. He's given little swabs of ice water to wipe his mouth—not much relief for being thirsty.

They stress using the breathing toy. He barely says a word. The words come in monotone and short phrases. He looks at me, but he is in another place.

When I arrive, he says he wants to shave. He's been waiting for me. "Oh?" I say, "Okay, what do I do?" I ask the nurse for his personal items and hot water. She seems busy and occupied. I get everything together, and the nurse finally comes over and says, "He didn't want me to shave him." She is worried that he will cut himself. He's on blood thinners. I'm caught in the middle and step back to assess the situation. Finally, it is agreed that Fred can shave with the nurse present, but he must be very careful not to nick himself.

She and I watch with anticipation at every swipe of the blade. Finally, he is satisfied. Later, when the nurse leaves, he says, "I doubt I would have bled.

She's just fussy!" I'm amazed—he's barely able to put a sentence together, yet his personality pushes through. Later he asks for pain medications; he's off the self-medication. The nurse asks about his pain level. They use a 1–10 scale, with 10 being the highest. He says, "1." She looks at him and says, "I can't give you pain medication for a 1. Are you sure?" I say, "He doesn't register pain like the rest of us. You and I would say it's an 8, and he would say he doesn't have any." She looks at Fred and says, "You can't have the operation you just had and not have a lot of pain. Now, what is it?" He says, "2." She asks again, "What is it?" And he says, "3."

They take his catheter out. He can't go. The nurse says, "That's ok, we'll just put the catheter back in." He goes right away—the trick of the nurse.

Monday, back to the floor. He goes for a Barium swallow to check if everything is holding. Looks good. He says he was gagging the whole time. He can drink now.

The new roommate is noisy and needy, calling the nurse every fifteen minutes and complaining about every little thing. He calls all his friends and relatives and tells each one every detail; he wants his wife to sit by his side every minute. Poor Fred, no peace.

Mom comes every day. It's nice to have company; we eat lunch together. She was worried and didn't want me to know.

Bonnie and Robear care for the animals; the winery is closed during the week, losing sales. I keep saying everything will work out somehow.

Tuesday: He starts soft foods. They take out the nose tubes. Everyone at the hospital looks familiar. Doug comes to visit and brings lots of magazines; only Fred can't read more than a few words without losing focus.

Wednesday: We go for two walks on the floor. I look at all of his incisions. The staples are huge; it looks like a shark attacked him. He has two major incisions: one from below the breast that zigzags around the belly button and goes down 4 inches (they accessed the stomach first during surgery). Then under the right arm and around to the middle of the back, they accessed the esophagus second, cut it out, and then pulled up the remaining stomach to attach to a little piece of the esophagus- a major reconfiguration of the digestive system. He still has to sit up 24/7.

Thursday: They take out the chest tube. I watch. It's two big tubes and another big hole in the chest. It burns for a while. He never complains. He has never complained about anything since this all began. He is brave. I have told my angel to stay with him. She has been doing double duty. The surgeon comes in, and Fred immediately says, "I want to go home."

Friday morning: Fred calls and says he can go home; they removed the staples.

I say, "I am on my way."

The Road Back

What a relief to be home! He has a feeding tube and lots of medications. But as we settle in, we realize this is all new, and we don't really know what to do.

I make Jello, mashed potatoes, and soft stuff. He tries to eat and says nothing. At night, he can't lie down. He ends up sitting up all night.

Saturday: They deliver the enteric feeding stuff. We set it up in the living room.

At night, he sits up again, going up and down all night. I wake up four times to move the feeding tube pole.

Sunday: He's exhausted because he couldn't sleep. I start checking things. I clean up the feeding tube hole. Incredibly, there's this gaping hole in his abdomen with a tube leading into his intestine. He doesn't eat again. Fifteen hours on the feeding tube for 1500 calories. We will try to start earlier.

Monday: At 4:00 p.m., the visiting nurse comes. I can tell she's assessing us very discreetly. She wants to wash her hands—oh well, things aren't that dirty. She examines each of Fred's incisions and takes out some stitches. The front incision isn't healing as well, especially around the belt line. She suggests some additional cleaning, demonstrates how to do it, and puts some extra dressing on. She asks Fred questions; he's polite, but I can tell he's impatient. I ask about a special pillow to help him sleep because he has to sit up. When she leaves, he says he doesn't want her to come back. I say I want her to come back, at least that week. He sleeps downstairs in a chair. I get the urinal out. The living room is becoming his room now. I check in the middle of the night for his breathing.

Tuesday is the same. He only drinks a little cranberry juice. He's captive with the feeding tube for 15 hours and not doing much during other times. He can't drive for three weeks and doesn't want to go outside because it's too cold. He tries to attach the feeding tube, but his hands shake too much, so I do.

Wednesday: He's very cold; the heat is set at 75 all night and day. I'm boiling. He wants me to eat in the kitchen because he can't bear someone eating around him. He tries some soup and throws it up. I buy all kinds of food. He doesn't eat anything, so I throw food out constantly.

Thursday: The nurse is coming. I wish Fred is back in the hospital. I don't know what to do or if I'm doing anything right. We go over the food menu they gave us. Fred wants to eat his food. He hates a soft food diet. For me, it would be fine. He eats a bologna sandwich and throws up. He hates the feeding tube. He is stubborn. Maybe he just doesn't feel well. If you looked like him, you wouldn't feel well.

The days drag on; I have to pick up the house, empty

the urinal, get drinks, and try lunch, and he doesn't know why he's no better. He can't sleep. He throws everything up due to reflux. We decide to insert the feeding tube during the day so that he can get up and down without dragging the pole all over the place at night. I sleep through the night. This is better.

He starts to eat a little, gets full quickly, and has reflux frequently.

The visiting nurse comes again, and she says it will get better. I agree with Fred not to have her come back.

He keeps trying foods that he likes. We've backed off the number of Osmolite cans/day to 1000 calories. I count the calories every day. Right now, a good day is 1,500 calories. That's not enough; he's losing more weight.

He's having half a sandwich and soup for lunch. He's full all day, tries some dinner, then throws up. He has reflux all night.

Every day is the same. He's losing more weight.

The days go on. We keep trying. I keep saying that this will get better. He won't take the nutritional drinks. I buy every brand on the market. He says he'll try. I review the calories in the Osmolyte and the calories in the nutritional drinks.

February 7, 2003

Friday: All the crises and big issues happen.

Finally, he says it's not working; he feels like he's starving and can't get enough nutrition. Is it psychological that he can't eat? Would you be afraid to eat if you lost your esophagus and half your stomach?

Monday: We prepare to call Dr. Goldberg. I make notes on the symptoms so I can communicate for Fred. Something's not right. He's full all the time and throws up every day.

Dr. G. asks a few questions. He says we should schedule him for another endoscopy. Most likely, the new stomach opening needs to be stretched. This is common. When? Tomorrow possibly, but we are seeing the heart specialist and would have to wait all day for the surgery room. Wednesday is scheduled.

At night, his feeding tube breaks loose. He pushes it back in, and we tape it up. But is it still in the intestine?

Tuesday: We leave early; Fred starts throwing up in the car. My thoughts are racing—what should I do? I call Rose, Dr. G's assistant, and leave a message. I think I made a mistake by waiting on the procedure. Fred is sick; can we still get scheduled today? Rose calls back before we get to the hospital. She says she will try and will call the heart specialist's office.

Fred gets a good report from the heart doctor; everything looks good, so he can reduce the medications. This is common. Fred says he's having a lot of problems and is nervous. The doctor says it's understandable; he's been through the war. It will take some time, but he will recover. The nurse thinks Fred's feeding tube opening is infected. I shudder at the idea.

Rose leaves us a message saying everything's scheduled for later that day. We go to day surgery at 11 a.m. without food—we know the drill.

I wait with Fred until they take him into the surgery room. Then I get lunch and sit again in the family waiting area. I just get settled when Dr. Goldberg comes out. This can't be good. We go to a private area, and I say, "That was fast!" He says it is when nothing is wrong. I'm not sure what that means. He stretched the opening, but it was already pretty good. Fred's stomach had noodles (from 24 hours earlier: a can of chicken noodle soup!) Dr. G says they are frequently surprised by what is still in the stomach. He says that I'm just going to have to tough it out; he thinks this will resolve itself over time and tells us to stay away from pasta. I remember a plumber telling me about pasta in garbage disposals and how it can clog them.

I'm relieved that nothing else is wrong. As I wait to see Fred, I start thinking, "Did I imagine this problem? Did I overreact? Is Fred hyper and causing this?" He is very nervous. He is also stubborn and won't eat the recommended diet. Frequent small meals and starting early in the day are not in his book.

Saturday, February 15, 2003

It's one week later–mid-February. On the fifth, my spine had an incident. I have an old, severe neck and lower back injury. I have more severe incidents that leave me unable to move. About a week ago, I was standing in the kitchen and turning to go to the fridge when it felt like Teutonic plates were sliding within my lower back. When that happens, it's bad. I grabbed a whole muscle relaxer. I usually only take ½ in the evening since it knocks me out. Two hours later, I'm still standing, and nothing is relaxing, so I take another and start moving upstairs. I know the drill: lie flat in bed. Of course, it's the weekend. I tell Fred not to worry; I'll probably be OK in the morning.

Three days later, I haven't moved.

Fred has been calling our doctor, who isn't in, and the backup won't prescribe anything since I haven't been there in over a year. Fred persists, and somehow he finds the strength. We're a pair—he's living on a feeding tube and has to sit up 24/7, and I'm upstairs in bed, unable to move.

I call Mom and say we need help. "Is Fred eating?" she asks. I have no idea. She comes on Tuesday. They get the doctor to prescribe the steroids, and Mom gets Fred something to eat. I haven't eaten in a few days. I don't think Fred has either; he really can't care for himself. After two days of aggressive steroid use, I feel better and can sit up. By Friday, I'm standing. The steroids make you think you can do anything. On Saturday, I walk downstairs. That's the fastest I've ever recovered. The key is getting the steroids immediately. I don't want to know about the side effects. The taper is after four days, and I don't feel as well, but I'm functioning.

We keep working on a diet that works. It appears to be better at first following the endoscopy, but then we sink into the same pattern. I keep saying it will get better. We just have to let time pass and look at the week-to-week or month-to-month progress. I'm pruning the vines as much as possible. We're having heavy snows this year—three feet high, up to the cordon wire. The snow piling up on the roof causes a leak in the new building. I have to get Fred to help me. He staggers around, barely able to gather his strength; just walking about in the snow and mush takes effort. He holds the ladder. I climb onto the roof with a big broom to remove the snow. We work together. He is exhausted.

The days go on. There's no visible improvement. I keep looking for signs that maybe it's getting better. The month is half over; the trip is in March—what will we do?

Keep going day by day. Fred is quiet. He is naturally a quiet person with strong Finn characteristics: happy to be alone, very strong and capable, and able to accomplish things alone. He can't understand why others need others so much. Except now.

Saturday, February 22, 2003

Four weeks until vacation. We talk of a possible plan to get there. Fred says he doesn't understand why this is not working. He's full all the time, has reflux all night and has to sit up most nights. Thank God we got the La-Z-Boy. He throws up half the time. He's still on the feeding tube but can now attach it himself. His hands still shake, but it's better. I patiently watch as he struggles to make the attachment. It reminds me of watching a fuel hookup in midair.

I talk to Dr. Goldberg. Something doesn't seem right. He asks new questions. He says it should resolve—if he doesn't have cancer brewing elsewhere! Fear rips through me. He says that sometimes he sees this happen if cancer develops in another area. We must find out if that's the case. I'm silent, steeling myself for another problem. We discuss tests and decide on a Barium swallow first. I decide not to tell Fred about the other possibility.

Thursday, March 6, 2003

The Barium Swallow: His stomach is full; the pyloric valve is shut, but something is leaking through. The pyloric valve is at the bottom of the stomach. The valve at the top is gone from the surgery. That's why the reflux so easily continues, maybe for life. Dr. G says that the pyloric valve can be fixed by surgery. They know about it, and he has a test he performs during the esophagectomy. They'll leave it alone if he can put his thumb through the valve. Fred's is okay. This rarely happens. Fred can't stand the feeding tube or the whole situation any longer. He wants it fixed. Dr. G. tells me okay, but he needs to ensure that something else—another cancer—isn't brewing. Again, I reset. I won't tell Fred. We discuss this procedure and the timeline. I'm still hoping to go on vacation. I'm hoping that this will be resolved soon.

Friday, March 7, 2003

We discuss the operation, and Fred is anxious to have the eating, being full, and throwing up problems disappear. I don't know what to do anymore. It doesn't seem right, but maybe something else is happening. I remain in purgatory.

Saturday, March 8, 2003

Fred says he wonders if this is too fast of a decision. I say maybe. We decide to get more information and call other doctors we know. Who will consult with us? I call Dave Hoffman, MD, a fellow grape grower, and Cynthia Baughman's husband, Jim. I have been working closely with Cynthia on the USAIR Attache magazine article.

Sunday, March 9, 2003

I call both doctors and leave messages. They call back later. Whenever I tell someone about Fred's cancer, I start crying. I rehearse and think I'm ready, but I always start crying. It makes me feel like it's just starting all over again. We discuss the pyloric valve, its function, and other related issues. Diabetic patients have this problem. An option is to go the conservative route and see what happens. I tell Fred about these things. It is another surgery, and there is a recovery.

Monday, March 10, 2003

We go for the first CT scan since surgery. We wait all day at Fox Chase to see Dr. G. He says the scan was "whistle clean." Good news. Now we have to decide about surgery to open the pyloric valve. He asks Fred what he wants to do. Fred needs time to decide. I inquire about any risks associated with the surgery. Dr. G says that the pyloric valve can become too loose, and stuff moves up from the intestine into the stomach. It doesn't sound like something we would be happy with. On the way home, Fred mentions that he was surprised that Dr. G seemed to be saying things differently today than last Thursday. I realize that Dr. G and I are both so relieved that nothing else appeared on the CT scan, and Fred didn't know we were worried about that. I tell him. He digests that and asks more about it. I say, "I didn't want you to worry more."

Tuesday, March 11, 2003

We discuss the operation again. I say, "Dr. G said it's possible that the pyloric valve will return to normal. It should, over time. Can you wait?" We would have to clean out the stomach and let things rest. One week on feeding tubes only, then restart the food. I call Dr. G and say, "We're going to try the conservative approach, and I told Fred this is like starting over after the surgery and to forget the last two months." Dr. G thinks that's a good idea—the starting-over concept. Also, he has been on the feeding tube only since Thursday because of the possibility of pyloric valve surgery. Liquids and pureed foods are OK.

Barbara brings over some nutritional drink flavors that she likes and recipes for pureed soups. She makes carrot soup. Fred likes it. I think he can just eat liquids and pureed foods for a complete diet. I work on lists of liquid meals. I explain to Fred that this is what we will do. He is skeptical and doesn't like that there is an end in sight. I say, "It will change, just give it a rest. Let's try it." He says yes, unenthusiastically. I have convinced myself that this will work. What a great solution... and I like these foods!

Wednesday, March 12, 2003

We discuss calories, nutritional drinks, pureed foods, and starting in the morning. He eats mashed potatoes at night with no reflux, small portions, and no feeding tube.

Thursday, March 13, 2003

We go out for an errand. We stop at the grocery store, but he can't go in. I buy more liquid stuff.

Friday, March 14, 2003

We talk about the trip; we're not sure yet and haven't told our travelling friend. I call the resort. I start crying when I tell Bruce at the dive resort about the cancer. Every time, it's the same. He doesn't know about diving with a feeding tube, but he suggests that DAN (Divers Alert Network) will know. DAN has medical staff on call. They are very helpful and say, "Yes, one can dive with an intestinal feeding tube." It's actually an air cavity in the body. We discuss ways to cover it up while in the water. It's unbelievable that you can dive with a hole in your abdomen.

Fred is more optimistic but doesn't want anyone to see the feeding tube. I can think of several ways to camouflage the feeding tube.

Saturday, March 15, 2003

Beware the Ides of March.

One week to vacation. He's much better about the food routine but still hates the nutritional drinks. We found one—Boost Tropical Fruit—that he'll drink in the morning. It has a calorie count of 160.

He occasionally eats a donut with 100 calories for a plain donut and 360 calories for a crème-filled donut. I push the crème filled. Lunch is pureed soup. He's eating 1500 calories per day and hasn't used his feeding tube in a few days.

Sunday, March 17, 2003

I give Fred the breakfast drink. Getting up is not fast. Later, he calls me upstairs. He says he wants to take out the feeding tube. This feeding tube has been the bane of his existence since surgery. But if it comes out and he still needs it, it will be another surgery. We discuss his present situation. I support his decision but remind him that he needs to continue the soft foods, expecting a gradual improvement. No McDonald's and bologna sandwiches! He agrees. We prepare to pull out the tube. It feels a little like the start of chemotherapy and our toast to the killing of the alien. I clean the area extra well and check just inside the opening. We have been taping it in place to keep the string from breaking again. Now we cut the string, and Fred pulls it out. It's a long, thin plastic tube. I ask if he feels anything; he says not much and nothing like pulling out the chest tubes. We clean the outside, remark on the size of the hole, bandage it up, and give each other the high five. Vacation is becoming more likely.

Monday, March 18, 2003

I'm busy preparing for our first PA Premium Wine Group meeting. This is Fred's baby, and I am the president; he's the treasurer.

I call our friend Mark Wagner. He's going on the trip with us. I have to tell him about Fred. Again, I cry. Will this ever end? I apologize for the last minute, but explain that Fred didn't want anyone to know, and we hardly told anyone. Now people are beginning to know. We're sorry this will impact him. Our trip will be different, and I want him to be prepared. He says we shouldn't worry about him; he's concerned for us. We talk about talking more.

Mark calls later, saying he was in shock earlier and wants to know more. He may try to visit this week; he lives 4 hours away.

Thursday, March 20, 2003

Preparations are ongoing. We pack many food items, the gear for snorkeling and diving, and a few clothes. Things get harder and slower as the day progresses. By dinner, I can barely move. At night I tell Mom I'm unsure if this is a good idea. Am I totally nuts to think we can do this? She says we've been planning and preparing, which will carry us through.

Friday, March 21, 2003

I got practically no sleep, worried about what I've forgotten, what I will say to people, and how others will act. I am walking around in circles, forgetting everything. It's a good thing I've been collecting things all week. I take Tashie to the dog spa. Finally, I finish packing. Our flight isn't until noon, so there's some last-minute time.

March 22-29, 2003

It's twelve weeks after surgery, and unbelievably, we are vacationing in Bonaire with a friend. This trip was planned over a year earlier, much before we knew of Fred's illness. The trip had become a goal of sorts. After the initial diagnosis, when we could finally ask questions, we began to ask about the possibility of going on this dive trip–7 months in the future. Fred always asked me to check with the various doctors. We asked the surgeon who installed the port under his skin, the thoracic surgeon, the medical oncologist, his nurse, and the radiologist. Every time our visit discussed a schedule, we asked. The doctors believe that travel is generally good for patients. It helps with the overall quality of life.

I would mention this trip to various people who were supporting me, and most would say, "You'll have to cancel that." But my instincts said that this trip was Fred's anchor to life in the future.

So we planned.

And we went.

We arrive late Saturday night, and travel wasn't too bad, just two flights from Philadelphia. I ordered special services, but Fred doesn't want any help. I brought special drinks and food; half our suitcase weight is drink supplements, soups, and cheeses— things that can form a routine. By now, we have tried every available nutritional drink, pureed soup, soft food, and supplemental food. I have memorized the calorie chart; anything worth more than 100 calories per serving is considered. Breakfast is a drink with 160 calories; a donut with crème filling is best at 250– 300 calories; lunch is 2 cups of pureed broccoli soup with 160 calories; and a sandwich with 400 calories. Lemon-lime soda, midafternoon, at 160 cal. The goal is 1,000 calories by midday. Cheese at 4 p.m., 300–600 cal, then dinner. Often a filet, 600–800 calories, maybe soup again, and some vegetables. Dinners are about 1,000 cal. Desserts aren't appealing. If we work at it, he can take in about 2000 calories per day. Tropical drinks in the late afternoon help with the calories and appetite for dinner. He has to sit up for a while most nights, but then he can lie down.

We get food for the day on Sunday and set up our kitchen routine. We rent the equipment for diving. Usually, on the first morning, we would go by ourselves for a check-out dive. There's a beach out front. Fred takes the gear out front, and we struggle to get it all set up; then, miraculously, he carries his tank down to the water and walks in. In shallow water, he tries to get into his dive gear and get his fins on. I pretend to get my gear together while watching. Finally, he starts to drag his gear out, half falling over. I run down to help and pick up the dive gear and tank, all the while talking about how slow I am to get my stuff together. We get him back in the water, and I join him. We snorkel out to sea, and then I try to submerge. My ears adjust slowly to pressure, so we have a routine where I go down 10-15 feet and signal when stable, and he descends. Then it usually takes forever, but eventually, we can descend to whatever depth we want. This day, however, I provide comic relief for us and everyone watching. I repeatedly try to go down in various ways—feet first, head first, swimming down—but I keep bobbing back up. Finally, we swim back to shore and get more weight for me, and then I am able to descend. By now, we have both gotten used to this unnatural act of diving. Later, we are relieved to have the first dive over; that is all we can do today. Fred says it was strange; I ask, "How so?" He says he was afraid; I say, "Now you know how I feel."

He has never admitted to being afraid.

Monday, March 30, 2003

Home feels good. We both resume our normal activities: unpacking, shopping, animal makeup time, and pruning the vines for me. He just can't do that this year. I still think about how great the trip was. We are renewed. It was a wonderful break. Fred's out and about. Finally, we have turned the corner.

Tuesday, March 31, 2003

Fred isn't feeling well. We talk, and he says he knows he hasn't been engaged in life since his diagnosis. He wants to re-engage, but all he thinks about is cancer.

Everything starts crashing in again. I can't move. I feel buried alive, but I have to keep moving.

Saturday, April 5, 2003

Bagdad is liberated. Fred is living in his own personal hell. No appetite (afraid to eat?), nauseous at the thought of food, depressed, afraid to get up in the morning–he's a mess (and says so)–a downward spiral. When will it end? Is this the grief that he didn't finish? He keeps everything in. I wonder if a P.O.W. would change places.

Wednesday, April 9, 2003

Fred's Birthday: He doesn't, can't, and won't acknowledge this day. He is deep in depression and has barely been able to get out of bed this past week. He is exhausted, has no appetite, is afraid to eat, and is fearful of what the day may bring. I think and say, "We will just get through today. Think only about today. Don't worry about the future—you can't control it." I wonder if this is the right thing to say.

Tuesday, April 15, 2003

Tax Day is not good for Uncle Sam this year, and it is not good for us either.

Fred was up at 2:00 a.m. He can't sleep, and his appetite is worse when he works. He stopped the Ritalin on Sunday; it made him a little hyper, and his appetite worsened. The pharmacist says that may be contributing to both sleep and appetite problems. Dr. Goldberg suggested Megace if he was still having a problem. They give that to AIDS patients who are wasting away. Tomorrow I'll call. We're just throwing drugs at poor Fred, hoping something will work.

Wednesday, April 16, 2003

Three and a half months after surgery: Everyone says he looks good. They convince themselves that he is OK. He's not.

Recovery is not like anything else. One can't just go out and do it, be tired, and get up the next day, like an exercise program that builds you up. I thought that would work. But it doesn't. This is different, I finally realize. It must be a new phase we're in, or I'm in. Maybe the caregiver has different phases. I should name them.

Saturday, April 19, 2003

My sister Kathy, husband Rick, and their son Tyler come to help me do hard labor in the vineyard—the replanting of Chardonnay and Gewurztraminer. Kathy brings lunch. We have a good time chatting. Fred can't get out of bed. He comes down, gets his lunch, thanks everyone, and looks like he will cry.

April 20, Easter Sunday, 2003

Fred is terrified when he awakes. He says he took some Percocet at 5:00 a.m. "Why?" I ask him. "I can't sleep; the painkillers worked in the hospital." I say seriously to him: "Painkillers work for pain; you were in physical pain in the hospital. Now you're in mental and emotional pain. You need to get up; don't stay in bed; it's not going to get any better. You need to dig deep and deal with this. Get up and do something; it will take your mind off this. Drugs are not going to do it. This is going to go on for the better part of a year; you need to figure out how you're going to handle it. You can't stay in bed all day." He says, "Maybe I'll stop taking the antidepressants; I don't know if they're doing anything."

I say, "I'll support you in whatever you want to do, but you need to decide how you'll handle it if you go into a panic, like the last time you went off medications. You decide and let me know."

I hope this wasn't too harsh; it felt like the right time to push. Maybe he's ready to break through; I know that can be scary.

Terrified in the morning with the first light of day
The sun is no longer a smiling friend
The fear of facing a new self

Unable to be as before

The fear that this is the new self

Poisoned forever

No strength

No focus

No joy

Monday, April 21, 2003

Fred's very depressed. He finally says he thinks he's afraid to go for the doctor's appointment on Wednesday, afraid of what they will say. This is with Dr. Cheng; we haven't seen him since before surgery. How does he interpret the results? The biopsy of the lymph nodes revealed live cells; I don't know how many there were and wish there were none. We may never know. I review all the positives with Fred, being careful not to say, "The cancer is gone." There's a patient who, eight months after surgery, is just eating solids. I tell Fred. Perspective helps.

I'm in a downward spiral. I thought this was over; it's been a while since I was overwhelmed with depression. Was I fooling myself? I feel so low and hopeless; will there ever be joy in my life again? I'm concerned about still being unemployed. Looking back, I have made some bad decisions and left a good job because of promises by a relative. I left a good retirement, health benefits, and salary. Now I have nothing. The annuity from 22 years of working for IBM only pays for our health insurance and a few bills. I feel desperate.

Maybe I'm feeling sorry for myself.

Fred has faced death,

There is nothing else to fear.

When he looks in the mirror, what does he see?

Tuesday, April 22, 2003

Fred can't eat today; he's too worried. I want to believe that the worst is over, but there is the possibility that something else is brewing. It's hard.

Wednesday, April 23, 2003

We go to Fox Chase early to get blood work. They are

not busy today. I go to the Y to swim and then meet Fred. He won't eat, so I take him to the snack shop to get something for later. While we wait for Dr. Cheng, he finally eats half the sandwich. There are so many people with cancer. We need to have patience. Finally, they call us; their scale is wrong; it says 200, while at home, it says 186.

Dr. Cheng asks, "Relative to one month, how do you feel? What about two months?" Fred talks about how he doesn't feel good, has no appetite, is very tired, can't sleep, and feels worse than he did two months ago. "What is the priority?" Fred can't separate. "Any bowel problems?" Some diarrhea. He reviews the current drugs. He talks about helping with some of those things but says that the main difficulty he sees is the emotional one. He says there are appetite aids like Megace to try first. But he says again that the main issue now is for Fred to take control of the situation. Fred asks, "Why am I so tired?" His hemoglobin is 11.7! Very good! It's returning already. They don't know why it sometimes takes so long to recover. They mention an NFL player who needs time off after the season because he is so beat up. "You had a very bad and large cancer that was advanced. We gave you the maximum treatment we could and did not kill you. Each of the treatments needs recovery, and together, it sometimes takes a year to recover. Think only of improvement on a month-to-month basis. You will return to how you felt before." He says that, unfortunately, Fred's cancer may come back, but they hope for a cure. No sense worrying; the doctors are optimistic, and new ways of treatment are coming. They will deal with it if it happens.

And then he says they see patients dealing with this situation in three ways:

1. They communicate and talk with people, not about the cancer but about other things.
2. They become active, either physically, like walking or running, even if they're tired, or by having activities.
3. If they are religious, they turn more to their religion to find hope.

Dr. Cheng says, "You need to decide what you are going to do to cope with this, and some people get divorced; that's how they deal with this." I know why.

He tells Fred, "I think you know what to do." Fred asks about a prescription for the other sleeping pill.

I wonder what he has heard.

April 24-26, 2003

We haven't talked about the doctor's visit. Fred is quiet. I got him Lance Armstrong's book, and he is actually reading it. He hasn't been able to read more than a page since this began. He goes out each day and does what he can. He's not getting stronger.

Monday, April 28, 2003

I'm busy getting ready for the Philadelphia and Pittsburgh Wine Festivals. It's a big deal that we are invited with 100 wineries worldwide. I'm thinking that Fred won't be able to go. Jon and Barbara will go to PGH with me. Fred's doing more and trying to do more, keeping busier. He seems less agonized. He's always been physical; it hurts him not to have that now.

Saturday, May 3, 2003

We drive back from the wine festivals. It was a wonderful experience for us and me. What an honor to be there! I've gained some new insights and perspectives. Jon and Barbara, and I talk about the quality effort for the new wine group. Barbara thinks I should find work in a related field. Why don't the member wineries pay me—I'm doing valuable work? I agree, but I don't think the wineries are in a position to do that.

We talk about Fred a little, and I try not to discuss it too much. Everyone must be sick of hearing about it all these months. I tell Barbara that I told Fred that this illness has given him an opportunity to start over and be however he wants. He can reinvent himself, and everyone will accept him. Barbara says that's interesting, but it may overwhelm Fred, and he may feel it is too big a task. We talk about another way to say that Fred can choose how he wants to be with people and if he wants to pick up where he left off.

Tuesday, May 6, 2003

I keep thinking about the lively woman in Pittsburgh toward the end of the festival. As she leaves our table with her husband, she leans close to me and says, "Something good is going to happen to you." I am surprised and say, "Good? I need it." She continues with, "It will." I reply, "You don't know how much I need it." She replies, "Oh, I do!"

I hope she's right. Just thinking about this conversation makes me hopeful. I am more positive that things will work out. I tell Fred, Kathy, and Nancy, my sisters, about this. I want them to know, and then I can tell them later when something good happens.

Wednesday, May 7, 2003

Fred is not so nervous. I say, "We haven't talked in a long time. Let's check-in." I think he appears to be less in pain and sleeping better. He says that is only outward. I ask about appetite. He doesn't think there is any improvement, but he's holding his own via the belt method. (What hole on the belt?)

We go to see Dr. Z, the psychiatrist. He says Fred

looks good. Everyone says that. Fred says he was thinking of something to talk about today. I'm pleasantly surprised; this is the first time. He says he can't enjoy anything, like a beautiful sunset. He looks at it and thinks about cancer. He says he knows he's a "glass is half full" guy, and he can't sleep past 4:00 a.m... If only he could sleep until 6. We discuss the medications, new possibilities, and combos to try. We discuss the increased activity and how that helps because our minds can only think of one thought at a time. So, anything to take your mind off the dwelling is good. Fred says he read a book. And then Z says that's significant. Four months have passed since the surgery. He talks about how there are many signs that things are improving, again stressing that it will be gradual. I ask about chemical depression, and he explains that when someone is depressed for a while, and this illness makes it very understandable how that would happen, the depression becomes chemical and feeds on itself. The neurons are frayed and need to be replenished. This will happen over time. The drugs can break the cycle. When we leave, I say, "Things are looking up." I remind Fred of what I said last week: that he is no longer the man who sees the glass half empty, but now he is the man who sees the glass half full.

Friday, May 9, 2003

I don't feel so desperate. I remember the woman in Pittsburgh. Something will work out. I have always believed this and that I should just stay focused on what I can do. Little by little, that's how we have built the winery. But I don't know what possessed me to believe we could succeed. Everyone knows that small wineries don't make any money—"It's a lifestyle," we say—even with winning a gold medal in Paris. Some things are changing, but we're still in Pennsylvania. That accomplishment would have caused a tremendous stir if we were in California. We can't even get the regional press to cover it! Secretly, I have always hoped and planned that it would support us. But the sad truth is that it doesn't yet and won't for many years. I have invested my life's fortune; why was I so sure we could do this against all odds? Now it seems like a careless gamble.

Monday, May 19, 2003

Fred is doing much better. He was able to participate in the winery's Spring Fling event and talk with a few people. His speech is a little slow, but everyone says he looks good! Ha!

He awakes and doesn't talk of the terror. He is more and more active and re-engaging. Finally, are we now survivors?

Wednesday, May 21, 2003

It has been one month since our last visit to Fox Chase. As we drive to the entrance, Fred says, "Back to the House of Horrors."

Blood work first, then we see Dr. Cheng.

The labs are good, except for the sugar level. Hemoglobin is 13! Dr. C. thinks the low sugar may be isolated and not relevant. We talk about the overall improvements. He sees improvement but is not yet back to pre-surgery levels, which takes time. He reinforces that Fred has been through the big one, the triathlon of cancer treatments. It doesn't get any bigger. I ask about possible insurance chemotherapy (this is still an unanswered question for me from a long time ago.) He says emphatically, "No. You couldn't take that. We gave you as much as possible to try to kill the cancer; we pushed the envelope, and you would not have gotten as much anywhere else in the country. Now we have to see if it worked." As we shake hands and thank him, he says we're doing good and should keep it up.

Thursday, May 22, 2003

In preparation for an interview, I have my hair cut. I talk about Tashie not feeling well. Bonnie encourages me to take her to the vet.

4:00 p.m. vet appointment: Tashie is jaundiced; they say she has a serious illness, possibly two things. I break down crying immediately, apologize, and say my husband has cancer, and it's been a tough year. Then I calm down and ask, "What do we do?" It's either a tick-borne disease or a liver disorder. I wait while they draw blood, thinking I will surely implode. I think of calling Bonnie and asking her to come sit with me. We have asked so much of our supporters. I don't have my cell phone. Finally, I recover my hospital waiting posture. Tashie is our most precious friend and companion. She is like our child. I can't call Fred. When is something good going to happen?

The blood results show a strong positive for Lyme disease. She seems stable, and they send her home to await more blood test results. I don't want to tell Fred. But I do. He is quiet and sad.

Friday, May 23, 2003

The vet says she has a very high bilirubin count. They're waiting for other test results, but Tashie should get an ultrasound asap. Finally, after many calls and back and forth, the specialist can fit us in now. I am leaving for my interview, so Fred must take her.

When I get home, there is a message from Fred. I can tell it is not good news. I call the vet, and Fred tells me that she has tumors in her bile duct that are causing the blockage. They are doing a chest x-ray to make sure there isn't cancer. Then Dr. Sadanaya will do surgery, and if the tumors are soft, he can make a bypass. If they are hard, that means cancer, and it is fatal. No, no, no. Dr. S wants to know what Fred wants to do in that case. I don't understand; Fred says that he asked if we wanted him to put her to sleep. Fred says, "No, wake her up, and we'll take her home. The blockage would eventually burst, and she would die."

This just can't be real. When is something good going to happen?

I hurry to the specialist, but they are working on her. I don't get to see her. We wait for another eternity. As time progresses, we get a little hopeful. It means that the surgeon can do the operation. Finally, after several hours have passed, Dr. S comes to talk with us. It is different than he thought, but he thinks there is no cancer, and he has done a very sophisticated bypass for the pancreas and the bile duct. She should make it; the next 24 hours are important.

Fred is exhausted. He says he has never experienced more trauma than today—worse than his situation. I ask if it was similar to learning he had cancer. He says it was different.

At night, Tashie is not sleeping with me. Fred sleeps in the La-Z-Boy.

Saturday, May 24, 2003

I am sad in the morning. Tashie's presence is missed. She fills our existence. I wait to call. Finally, I reach the technician; she is doing well; on IVs, the bilirubin is now 4.6 (it was 7.8; normal is 0 to 0.9).

Precious One

You shower us with joy,

By your companionship, your interest,

And your unconditional love.

You are lightness,

And playfulness, and fun.

You create brightness,

Just like the sun.

Sunday-Monday, May 25-26, 2003

We are waiting to hear more about Tashie. (Fred

writes her name as Tashy.) We hope that she will be OK. If she were better, that's as good as it gets.

Memorial Day

We barricade ourselves in. Tashie has to stay another day. Her bilirubin count goes up a little.

Tuesday, May 28, 2003

Tashie can come home. She is wearing a collar and can't jump into the car. At home, we take the collar off and vow to watch her. She doesn't seem interested in the incision but is just relieved to be home. She seems fine. We will wait for more info.

Friday, May 29, 2003

Tashie is doing well and eating. It is hard to keep her quiet.

I take her to get blood drawn in the morning. I ask about the biopsy results. Before I leave, Dr. Sadanaya wants to talk with me and see Tashie. He just got the results and is reading them in the room while talking to me. He says, "Oh no, she has pancreatic cancer." The words register, but there are no feelings. We talk briefly, and then I start crying and tell him about Fred. We discuss the treatment possibilities. The only hope is to prolong the cancer with chemotherapy. Her liver, however, must return to normal, or she will be unable to tolerate the chemotherapy. I can't believe this is happening. What will I tell Fred, and how will I tell him?

Oh God, where art Thou?

Surely on vacation.

It's Ten Days Later

I could barely talk to anyone. I'm walking on eggshells. We have seen the local veterinary oncologist. Our veterinarian tells us that the specialist is always very optimistic. We should know what our goal is. I tell her that we know that in humans, pancreatic cancer is not curable today. She says it's the same in dogs.

We go to the veterinary specialist; she is very optimistic and talks about the national cancer conference she just returned from. There is a lot of talk about Gemzar and pancreatic cancer. They can now extend human life by up to ten years. That's two years in dog years. She talks about the early diagnosis; she's never treated this before, and the cancer is always so advanced when the vet sees the animals, similar to humans. We leave feeling optimistic and plan to begin chemotherapy immediately with seven weekly or biweekly $500 treatments. Then there will be an ultrasound; if there is no growth, she will continue chemotherapy every three weeks for up to six months, followed by an ultrasound every two months. Tashie could resume her normal life if there is no growth by the end of chemotherapy. We would be happy with a few more years.

In my brain, I hear the cautionary words of our local vet; the specialist is very optimistic. Usually, I am ready to sign up right away, and Fred wants to think it over. This time, I say, "We want to think it over." In the car, Fred asks why I didn't want to start immediately. I say, "For two reasons: 1. You usually prefer to think it over, and 2. I remember our vet's caution."

I have been thinking about calling Fred's oncologist about this drug. He will surely know about the treatment in humans. The next day, he returns the call, but I am not home. Fred says he didn't do well on the phone with Dr. Cheng. He got confused and can't remember much. These confusion and memory loss have been exacerbated since the chemotherapy and/or radiation. I call Dr. Cheng again, and when we talk, he is not hopeful. He was at the same national conference as the veterinary specialist. If this drug could prolong the patient's life for ten years, that would be very big news, and everyone would be talking about it. He is current on all work in that area and would know. He says chemotherapy alone will not cure pancreatic cancer or prolong it for over a few months. I say, "But this is very early; there are no symptoms, and nothing is showing on the ultrasound." He repeats to me that chemotherapy will not do very much alone. Chemotherapy and radiation can help, and it's better if the cancer is extracted. He asks if the tumor was removed. No, it was too hard to get. OK, then we can do radiation? It is very expensive for animals. He is sorry to have to tell us this. He can't advise us, and I say, "We know, but we trust you, and we knew you would know about the treatment." "Would you treat your dog?" I ask. "No," he says. "There is stress and side effects, and the results are minimal. "Thank you, Dr. Cheng, for talking with us.

I call our local vet to ask for help. I am confused and very sad.

I am getting ready for the Wegman's wine festival. We need to leave by three. We have to keep moving. Fred is coming today and will help me set up. It's probably too much for him, but he will try. Before we leave, Dr. Leslie, our vet, calls, and I tell her about the meeting with the veterinary oncologist and then about the conversation with Dr. Cheng. I read the biopsy report to her and tell her that Dr. Cheng says this is the garden variety of pancreatic cancer, which is not very treatable. She is very sympathetic and realizes we have a lot going on. I am crying again and trying to tell her what I know. She immediately takes on the role of helping us get another opinion about chemotherapy. She will talk to the oncologist at Penn's vet school.

Later, I tell Fred about the conversation. We are destroyed, torn, and used up. He says that now we know why some people give up—it's just too much to bear.

I travel to Allentown for the festival on Friday, Saturday, and Sunday. Jon goes with me on Saturday and helps with the seminars we are putting on. I call Fred after dinner and give him a report. It has rained all day, and the crowds are smaller and more interested than the Friday night "let's get drunk" crowd. "How is Tashie?" I am crying again. Fred tries to comfort me and tells me how sad he is, and he wants to cry, too. And he doesn't know what to say when I say I don't know what to do anymore. He says we will get through this somehow. This is the first time since he was diagnosed that he has comforted me. It must be the next phase.

Monday, June 9, 2003

I am exhausted from the three days of the festival. We poured about 1000 tastes per day. Sales were minimal. Most of the attendees are there for a good time and to get drunk. I hate this about wine festivals in this state. Mostly, you see arms held out in front of you, sticking their glass at you and saying, "Gimme some of that." I reply, "Sorry, what did you want to taste?" This was a Breast Cancer benefit.

Fred tells me that Dr. Gail, the vet, called on Saturday and spoke with the oncologist at Penn, who advised not to treat. Confirmed. Now we know. I cancel the chemotherapy appointment.

I remember the paragraph I keep returning to in Lance Armstrong's book. About why people are so afraid of cancer: it is a slow and painful death.

Tuesday, June 10, 2003

We see Dr. Z in the afternoon. I think that I will talk about how I feel about Tashie. We're busy; my brother Paul has been over to help with the frontscaping. He does beautiful work, but he can't function very well since his botched brain surgery. It may be his new reality. Fred starts talking with Zubie. Fred always looks good; everyone always says so, but now he is starting to look more alive. He's gained back a few pounds and has good coloring. He tells Zubie about Tashie, and I start crying. I've always hated that about girls in movies who cried at everything. They talk about

Fred's status. Zubie says it's been five months since surgery—we thought we'd never get there. He says that it's time for Fred to be normal again, that things will return to normal, and then we will forget that everyone thinks they'll hold each day special, but as time goes on, it does return to normal. I listen while they talk and watch Fred. Finally, I say that I can't believe that things will ever be normal again. Nothing is the same. We talk about resuming relationships and telling Fred's parents. Zubie encourages Fred to tell his parents sooner than later. It's time now, and it's actually a putdown not to tell them. Fred says he's been thinking about telling them, OK. When we leave, I tell Fred that I can barely stand all the sadness because of Tashie; I feel like I will surely break into little pieces, and how can anything ever be normal again? He says he feels the same. I say, "We're nicer to each other now, and I want that to stay the same." He says, "Me too." We hold hands. I look at his hair and marvel at the black hair coming in, which is thicker and curlier. I tell him how nice he looks. He squeezes my hand.

Wednesday, June 11, 2003

It's hot for a change. The weather has been wet, wet, wet this spring, and cool. This is the first week of seasonable warmth. And the sun has been mostly absent. The state viticulturist says the weather is Oregonish.

We sit in the living room and talk about Tasthie.

I am trying to get a job, hoping something good will happen.

Saturday, June 14, 2003

Fred's had a rough night and doesn't feel well. Mostly he's doing well, and the off days are more infrequent. We decide to disgorge champagne tomorrow.

Fred just came to get me, and Tashie's been barking for ten minutes at the top of the vineyard. We rush out—it's usually because she has a groundhog cornered. If they're too big, we have to go and assist in the kill. She was bitten by one as a puppy and has never forgotten it. Every year, she gets at least a dozen and parades them around. This was a small one, but in the brush. She's a mighty hunter.

Sunday, June 15, Father's Day 2003

We disgorge champagne. Fred is able to do a complete batch. I notice he has faded about 65% of the way, but he hangs in there, just like old times. I finish up, and he goes back to the house. A few hours later, I check on him, and he has crashed, can't eat, and is overdone. I am busy in the winery with more USAIR Attache Magazine article customers. His daughter calls, but they don't connect.

Monday, June 16, 2003

I'm still recovering from the festival and can't do what I could at 30. I have to work smarter. Fred is still overdone. I realize that he hasn't been eating well. I've been busy and need to pay attention again. It's always an effort to make sure he eats enough. He wants to eat "normal" food. Anne can't believe he can eat as much as he described in one sitting. He wants to eat Oreos, a whoopie pie, or ice cream after dinner, but every time he tries, he has reflux for half the night. Sometimes it's so bad that I have to leave the room. I try to act like everything is normal, but it isn't.

Wednesday, June 18, 2003

Tashie is still doing well, with no signs of deterioration. Fred and I don't talk about it. Fred picks up her biopsy slides.

Sunday, June 22, 2003

The Summer Solstice. Now things will be better. The rain has stopped. I am in so much pain that I can't stand up. I take more cyclobenzaprine and lay down on my stomach. Later, I get up and am better. I visit several gardens on the local garden tour and go to the pool.

After dinner, Tashie comes into the living room but can't get comfortable. She keeps moving and starts to lie down but sits up and hangs her head. I hug her on the floor, and she leans her body against mine. We stay like that for several minutes. Fred watches. I am thinking this is the first sign of change. Fred makes a spot on the footrest of the La-Z-Boy. She curls up on the footrest, leaning against Fred, and keeps her head up for a long time. Fred pets her head softly, and she finally closes her eyes and lays her head down. She stays like that all evening until we go to bed. Sadness takes over.

Fred's been coming to bed in the middle of the night the last couple of nights. He's trying to get back to "normal."

Monday, June 23, 2003

The sun is out, and it's a beautiful day. Finally, after two months of cloudy weather, I can work on my to-do lists in my office space. A traveling salesman stops to see if we want our old barn roof painted. We were planning to do so this year. We discuss and look at pictures, ask for references, and in the end, we say yes because we believe there are still honest people. They arrive in 30 minutes and start the power washing.

I am out to the pool at 5 p.m. and return home after the start of the evening news. I am hand-feeding

Tashie when I hear the headline for the next story about a doctor at Brigham and Women's Hospital in Boston who has cancer—esophageal cancer. "This is one of the deadliest cancers, with 80% of patients dying within five years."

Fred goes pale. We have never asked for the statistics. The doctors always skirt around the statistics. I tell him I know he will survive. We talk for an hour. Fred asks if his cancer can come back. I say yes. The same questions keep coming up. His esophagus is gone, so he can't get that again. He could get stomach cancer again, and then they would take the rest of his stomach. And then... But I say that 80% is the national average. He says, "Yes, the national average, and I'm an average patient." But, I say, "You went to Fox Chase to increase your odds, and they wouldn't have taken you if they didn't think you could be cured. After all, they don't want their statistics dragged down." This is supposed to make him feel better.

Thursday, June 26, 2003

We go back to Fox Chase to see the radiologist. Fred

says I don't have to go, but I say I want to while I can. I clean up after the roof painters. There are zillions of tiny paint chips everywhere.

On the way to the hospital, Fred is very animated, more like his old self. He's excited and forceful in telling me what I should have told the new PA Wine Assoc. president I talked to earlier in the day. I have my own approach. Fred has previously criticized my approach, calling it too wimpy and not straightforward, and says I should tell them the truth. I listen and wonder why he is so riled up.

Dr. Konski sees Fred when we get to the receptionist and says, "It's good to see you." Fred says, "It's good to be here." He checks Fred's throat, glands, and incision areas. I am wondering what he will ask about, remembering Dr. Dave's comment about the longer-term negative effects of radiation. Fred talks about how he's feeling now. He looks reasonably relaxed and in control. He talks about the time before the last six weeks, the struggles, and how he feels the change in his recovery, the jump forward in the last six weeks. He can eat most of what he wants; there are limitations, and how he eats has changed, but he really has no complaints. He describes what happens if he eats the wrong thing or too late: reflux. They say everyone is different regarding what they can and cannot eat. You just have to learn what works for you. He's lost two pounds. Dr. K says that there will always be something to watch. I remind Fred to mention the lack of allergy symptoms this year. Dr. K believes this is due to the chemotherapy's effect on the immune system. I add the word "suppress" in my mind. Fred says, "I guess you couldn't sell chemotherapy and radiation as allergy treatments." Dr. K laughs. When we leave, he says, "See you next year." That's the first time someone at the hospital has said that. I try to reinforce that as we walk to the car. We smile, hold hands, and comment on how it feels like we were just let out of school, "Or prison," Fred says.

On the way home, it feels relaxed; we talk about how far he's come and how it is only five months from surgery. Five hard months. I say, "We forgot to tell Dr. Konski that he went scuba diving 2 ½ months after surgery. It's hard to believe we did it now." Fred says he wishes we hadn't. He was very uncomfortable the whole time. Even while diving, he couldn't think of anything else. He says that Dr. G told us he should be able to go; we asked all the time and right before surgery. I say, "They don't want to say you can't do something because it may be good for you." And for Fred, it may have been something he thought he should have been able to do, so it stayed a goal.

It occurs to me that Fred is very different now than during the ride to the hospital. He must have been anxious over the visit, even though there would be no news, or so we hoped

Sunday, June 28, 2003

I am thinking about this entry and remember that I was very uptight and anxious about everything last Tuesday and Wednesday. Maybe I was nervous about Fred's visit. Things are so often not what they seem.

Thursday, July 2, 2003

I have been embarrassed about Pastor Cindy's visit. I feel weak and vulnerable, and I should not be feeling sorry for myself. I have much to be thankful for.

I think we have come so far, one day at a time. Why doesn't the end seem closer? Sometimes I read the cards in the grocery store. I keep looking until I find one that says something to me. Today I bought this one so I could reread it:

I'll bet you've had about enough
Of people telling you how strong you are
And how great you're doing during
This awful, difficult period in your life.
Maybe you'd rather hear someone say
How much this sucks, how outrageous
And unfair it is.
Maybe you'd rather hear
Someone tell you that you don't
Have to be strong all the time.
Or that it's definitely OK
To curse fate and throw
A tantrum or two.
So here I am to tell you

All that stuff and more,

To let you know where I stand,

Which is right in your corner.

There's no right or wrong way

At a time like this.

However you work through this thing

Is immaterial to me.

All I care about is that

You ask for what you need,

Lean on those who love you,

And try to trust me when I say

That you'll come out the other side.

– JEANNIE HURID

I don't know who Jeannie Hurid is, but thank you for writing this.

Fred is definitely returning to normal. Today, I tell him he needs to practice some of his new skills in patience.

Monday, July 7, 2003

Fred has reflux during dinner. He says again that he ate too fast. Only a little came up, not the whole dinner. I'll have to do a calorie check; he's losing weight again, maybe just from the heat.

Saturday, July 19, 2003

I guess it is just from too much all around, but I have spent the last week recovering again from a serious back incident. We had all the medications this time, and I started taking them on day 2. It didn't seem as bad or painful at first, but it was in the severe category by day three. Also, I didn't experience a big lift from the steroids right away, which worried me at first. On Wednesday, I was going crazy, kept trying to get up, and finally did stand by late afternoon. The electric Neurostim machine is very important. On Thursday, I was able to get up in the morning, and by late morning, with the Neurostim machine constantly on, I made it downstairs. After 30 minutes, the Neurostim machine died, but miraculously I started to feel better standing and could finally feel the push from the steroids. I was able to stand up till around 4 p.m., then crashed. I spent the time talking to the medical company about a new Neurostim machine. The bottom line is they won't get it shipped that day, which means I won't get it till Monday because the overnight carriers won't deliver on Saturday to us for some goofy reason. It's a carryover from the last century when this area was actually sparsely populated.

Tuesday, July 22, 2003

Fred is doing well.

Fred just asked if I know about Pastor Cindy's other patient, Kurt. I say, "Yes," and he says, "Is it bad?" A moment's pause flashes through my brain. I say, "Yes—he's dead." Finally, it's out, and I am unemotional. We talk about it—when it happened and the fact that I decided not to tell him what I knew, which was that he died of some complication, one of the endless complications. Our doctors say it was not treatment-related. He glares at me to see if I am holding anything back, then gazes out the window. It's been over nine months since he talked to Kurt. Fred digests this; it must be a shock for him. I say that somehow our paths have crossed because, for some reason, we knew of Kurt. He has died; Fred has lived. I recall the many times I have heard of someone dying—a grandfather or uncle—and then a baby being born. It feels like that with Kurt, he has died, and Fred will live. He says it must have been upsetting for me to know this and asks if our friends know. "Yes, and yes, thank God for my supporters; I could not have borne this alone." We go over the outcome of his treatment repeatedly, as best we can. He says he's strong enough to take another round of chemotherapy. He's nervous and aware that his next CT scan is exactly one month from today. That will tell us our future for the next six months. He talks about the first CT scan after surgery and the "clean as a whistle" verdict and is trying to convince himself that it is meaningful for the future.

Saturday, July 26, 2003

The days are dragging on. I'm feeling well enough to get around but not well enough to make progress on any chores. I've been behind for two months; I'm used to this happening. It's depressing to be minimally functioning.

Fred has been spraying the vineyard constantly. We had two 2-inch rainfalls this week, which washed off all spray material. This season will separate the "men from the boys" in wine grape-growing land. He is now able to do what needs to be done to save the grapes. Only the weather gods know for sure this year. And then, at harvest, we will come to know the real winemakers—another opportunity.

Sunday, July 27, 2003

Stuck in a dark place,

Struggling to find the light.

I have sunk again to the bottom,

In search of myself.

I used to be so sure of myself,

Now I know nothing.

I always saw endless possibilities,

Now there are no paths.

No happiness,

No joy,

No dreams.

Where is the reason that was the drive?

My life has no motion.

Fred has faced death,

There is nothing else to fear for us.

Is that where the energy and will have gone?

I can't let him see my despair. I cry in the car, just like old times.

Monday, July 28, 2003

I realize that my recent foray into introspection may be tied to my birthday, which is tomorrow. I remember being self-critical just before my birthday—I'm a year older, and what have I accomplished? I feel better with that realization.

Saturday, August 2, 2003

Fred's tone is irritable and anxious; he is annoyed

and impatient. He's making me mad. I tell him he's being rude. We discuss a special wine order; he can't remember that we made these arrangements in April. He participated in the conversation but can't remember. This is a chronic problem, I think, from the chemotherapy drugs. I hope it will go away. Finally, he says he's going through a new phase; he's irritable and angry. I'll need to be patient.

He doesn't know why or won't say. He says he's not thinking about the upcoming CT scan.

Monday, August 4, 2003

Some days I don't write; desperation and despair are my sparring partners.

Sunday, August 10, 2003 – One Year Since Knowing

We walk together, laughing about our dull lives.

The days flow on,

Sunset is our friend,

We've made it another day.

Wednesday, August 13, 2003

Anne, Dr. Cheng's assistant, calls, and we chit-chat a little. I ask about the biopsy results from the surgery. We have never known. She reads Fred's reports and says there are three layers of lymph nodes that they take out. Level 1: 6 out of 8 live cells; level 2: 2 out of 4; and level 3: none or one, I've forgotten which. Level 3 is farther away from the tumor. Also, she says he had a small piece of rib six removed. That's a surprise.

Saturday, August 16, 2003

Fred's getting nervous and speaking in monosyllables again.

Sunday, August 17, 2003

He's too stressed to eat. We talk a little, and he takes an Ativan. He eats a little, and we go upstairs to rest and read. I tell him not to worry. Anne says hello and tells us that it's important that he's been making progress. That means everything is fine; nothing is brewing (hopefully).

He starts talking and says he has pain in his chest. I ask him where, and he points to the bottom of his rib cage on the right side. I tell him about the 6th rib removal in surgery. Then he tells me that this hurt the whole time in the hospital. He never said a word. The removal of the rib piece most likely causes his current pain. He's been using his right arm a lot with the green hoe, which probably aggravated it. I think he feels a little better and less worried.

Monday, August 18, 2003

I find him sitting in the living room, hunched over and wringing his hands. I've never seen him wring his hands before. I say, "You're ringing your hands; are you OK?" We talk for a few minutes, but I do most of the talking. It's going to be a long 48 hours until the appointment.

Wednesday, August 20, 2003

It's 2:30 a.m., and I can't sleep. Finally, we will know

our destiny for the next six months. It's like living with a ticking time bomb; you never know if the fuse has been detonated. I am preparing for a celebration tonight.

They didn't give us a get-out-of-jail-free card. The March CT scan showed a dark area on his left lung. They want to do another scan without the contrast dye and then possibly a biopsy. Anne tells us this while we wait. I get very nervous; this can't be good. Dr. Cheng wants to do a biopsy; he doesn't know what it is; it's either scar tissue or disease. He asks another radiologist to look at it, and she says it should be biopsied. Why bother with the CT scan when you can do the biopsy now? They can't get us on the schedule for two weeks. Dr. Cheng tells us what the treatment would be: surgery right away to cut it out, lots of diagnostic tests before; he runs through a list of things; we nod; we know. We're in shock, I forget to go to scheduling, and we walk out the door. It's been almost a year since this started, and it feels like it's starting all over again. I want to scream and cry, but I have to keep my composure for Fred. We must be stuck in another reality; this can't be happening.

We decide to drink the champagne anyway and toast ourselves for eternity at home, and Fred says it may be cut short. Then he asks, "Is this how it's going to be—they just keep taking pieces out of me?"

I think I will break into a million pieces.

Thursday, August 21, 2003

I call Anne to ask if she will follow up to get the schedule improved. She calls in the afternoon. I am frustrated and angry. I say, "It feels like we don't know what's going on; we just found out last week that he lost a piece of his right rib in surgery, and yesterday we found out there was an area of his lungs that showed inflammation on the March CT scan. Maybe these are nothing, but they make me feel like we don't know everything."

She tells me that once they have the biopsy results if it's diseased, we will go through a testing phase. They won't do surgery if anything else shows up. That means the cancer will have spread to multiple locations. Then what happens? They just do chemotherapy for as long as possible. I don't want to know this.

Later that day, Fred and I talk about what we know. Fred wants to be optimistic, saying that the cancer hadn't spread before his diagnosis, so there's a good chance it hasn't. Later, he says he thinks Cheng already knows and believes it's cancer. That's what he's preparing for. I ask, "How will we get through the next two weeks?" He says he's going to work as much as possible.

Friday, August 29, 2003

I can't write or speak to anyone. Yesterday, I talked with Dr. Cheng. It is unlikely that this 2-cm spot is not diseased. He agreed that it had grown quickly. It is either lung cancer or esophageal cancer that has spread. Most likely, it's the latter. He says those statistics we heard on national TV are correct: 80% of esophageal cancer patients die within five years. "Is it because this is what happens—it spreads?" "Yes," he says. I don't feel better, just more gloomy.

Sunday, August 31, 2003

My dear sister Kathy, I go to her pool to swim since,

for some reason, my Y always closes on Labor Day weekend. We talk a little on the ride there and more after swimming. I feel terrible emotionally. I don't know what to do—keep going along or go for a second opinion; maybe we should now go elsewhere for treatment. Maybe this is all Fox Chase can do for us. Maybe I should have been doing more research on alternative methods. Kathy says she thinks I should know that Fred is going to die. I ask, "Is that what everyone thinks in my family?" Slowly, she says no, but maybe it's better for me to have her say that. She asks if that is so terrible of her. I say, "No; I'm so sick of everyone acting like this is no big deal; he's over the hard part, and he'll just get better, like your friends with prostrate or breast cancer." They simply don't understand.

Fred may make it. This spot could be scar tissue; it's not likely, but there's still a chance. There's also a chance it's lung cancer rather than esophageal cancer; it's unlikely, but it's possible. And there's a chance there aren't any other spots, in which case they can just remove this one and he'll be fine. So I will try to do everything I can to help and encourage him, as hard as it is. And I will need a lot more help and support. My support network is narrowing to almost only family and a few close friends who are not afraid to go the distance.

They say that humans will be judged by how we treat our animals, and I think all other animals on this earth will be as well. I think we will also be judged by how we care for and support those among us fighting for their lives.

Faith, hope, and courage—we need these things. I pray for help in the highest order. Faith that some justice exists, hope for a future, and courage to face what's ahead.

September 1, Labor Day, 2003

I ask Fred how he is doing. "I'm afraid," he says. That's all he can say. I hold his hand.

Wednesday, September 3, 2003

Lung Biopsy. Fred has had diarrhea since Saturday. I'm tired of cleaning the toilets. He tells me that he doesn't have any more Immodium when we leave. I only go out at least once a day to get stuff for him and ask him if he needs anything three times per day. We may have to stop on the way to the hospital. He drives. We leave at 6:20 a.m., and I wake up at 5 a.m. to prepare. He gently swerves from the right side of the lane to the left. It's raining slightly. It's going to be a bad ride. I have to tell him to move over or brake about ten times. From his view, nothing is wrong; why am I picking on little things? I just want to get there alive. He says I will make him mad. I say, "Next time I'm driving." We spend the rest of the time in silence. He's mad. He has a right to be mad, just not at me.

I talk to Anne about his prescriptions and the diarrhea. She thinks it's probably nerves. They ask if he can stay still for an hour. They can give him Immodium. He says yes; he's not postponing the biopsy. I explain to the nurse that we've waited two weeks for the test and; we don't want to reschedule. I wait for hours for the lung biopsy to be completed.

Finally, they take me to the recovery room, where he's sitting up and looking relaxed. I say, "How are you?" He replies, "Fine, the doctor said it looked

like a benign tumor, but she's been wrong before."
I brighten with relief; there's some hope. Later, the doctor sees me in the hall and says he can go home after one more chest x-ray. Part of his lung deflated, so they're watching it. I ask about the appearance, and she says it looks like a calcified lesion, sometimes indicative of a benign tumor, but the biopsy is the only way to know for sure. As we leave, Fred is in the bathroom, and Dr. Cheng walks by in a group. I give him a little wave, and he waves back, then he asks if they did the biopsy. I tell him about the calcified part; he says that's maybe a good sign, and we'll keep our fingers crossed. We'll talk on Friday.

The gloom lifts; there is hope. When I gave Fred a pep talk yesterday, I told him I'd called in my one miracle for this life. The miracle is that he and Tashie are cancer-free now.

We stop on the way home at Burger King for a big whopper and fries for Fred. As we get closer to home, Fred says, "Pull over here," and drops his pants for a bout of diarrhea.

Friday, September 5, 2003

In the afternoon, I leave for errands and call Dr. Cheng. He asks if I would rather talk in person, and I say, "I guess that means it wasn't benign." He says, "The preliminary report says no." I ask, "How many patients that he sees like Fred does this happen to?" He replies, "About 50%." He says it's better to wait until the report is final, and we will talk on Wednesday about the options. I tell him I won't tell Fred, and he thinks that's wise. And also, says to take this one day at a time. That feels like a message to me. We hang up.

I start crying so hard that I have to pull over. I call Mom. She is trying to be optimistic. I say, "Mom, there's a lot of growing evidence right in front of me. I don't think there's anything to be optimistic about."

I try to push these thoughts out of my head. There is a possibility that he can still survive. We have to try. Maybe my miracle will happen now.

Monday, September 8, 2003

My mind is fighting; it is conflicted. I keep fantasizing about the worst. What will I do if Fred doesn't make it? Stop thinking like this; it's negative. How is he doing? He looks like he's wilting away. He still has diarrhea. Kathy thinks he looks sad. When I ask how he is, the answer is, "I'm scared."

Tuesday, September 9, 2003: Nighttime

I haven't called Dr. Cheng—we'll hear the final results together tomorrow, but I don't know if I can make it. It feels like I will crumble into a heap and melt away. I call Kathy. She asks, "Do you want Mom to go with you?" I reply, "Mom has too much on her mind; it must be too much for you too." Calmly, she asks about Fred and how I am doing. She talks calmly and listens. I say, "I don't know how I'm going to get through this. It feels like it's starting all over again. I will need a lot of support." She asks if I want her to come and stay with us. "That won't help Fred," I say. She says, "But it will help you." I say, "I'm thinking about that." Then she says, "Well, there is the unknown, and you've experienced that before. It's a roller coaster, and you've experienced that before."

I don't say that I'm afraid that things will deteriorate quickly with Fred; the whispers of past stories float around the edges of my brain.

The cancer spreads quickly.

They didn't know how long

3-4 years, maybe

And three months later, he's gone.

Wednesday, September 10, 2003: The next first day of the rest of our lives.

I'm busy working on my consulting project and getting things done, so I don't fall too far behind. Fred doesn't want to get blood work; he just had it, and we have to sit around the hospital for so long. We decide to skip it this time. He waits in the car while I swim at the Y on my way to the hospital. One mile every day. Sometimes I swim in the right lane, where there is some turbulence, so I can pretend I'm in the ocean.

We wait an hour before Dr. Cheng comes in to the exam room. I am getting frantic. Finally, he arrives and asks how Fred is doing. We discuss the diarrhea; he has lost 8 pounds in two weeks. He prescribes an anti-diarrhea medicine. Then he says the lung biopsy shows it's the same cancer—esophageal. He talks about treatment options. Surgery: Fred is still young and relatively strong. chemotherapy may or may not help before surgery. The real question is: has it spread elsewhere? This has probably been there for some time—before surgery, at least. Esophageal cancer is so bad because the cells move to another spot, take up residence, and change their environment, making it hard to kill them. Chemotherapy can get to the live cells in the blood system, but not when they have taken up residence elsewhere. So maybe the PET scan will show more detail—either confirm there is nothing else or show there is. If nothing shows up, maybe surgery now is best, and then we will wait to see if anything else shows up. I ask if Fred can still be cured, and Dr. Cheng says slowly, "Yes, but your chances are significantly reduced." Fred asks if this means the clock is reset—five years to be cured with no incidence—and says, "Yes." He says he's sorry to give us this news, but it's better to go after things head-on. We're supposed to see the surgeon right away. We leave numb.

Thursday, September 11, 2003

I'm in the city, starting project interviews. I called Jennifer, Fred's daughter, on Tuesday. We connect, and I tell her to come down for a visit; we got bad news yesterday, and Fred needs all the support he can get to help him keep fighting. She says she will work on it. I say, "Sooner than later." I'm not sure if she really heard me.

Sunday, September 14, 2003

We try to do, not think. We're living in limbo again. I fear the worst. Fred is becoming exhausted and is unable to eat or drink. Diarrhea prevails.

Monday, September 15, 2003

Fred follows up on the stool sample we took to the lab on Friday. There are no results by noon. I call our GP, and they just got the results: negative. They can treat him that day, but they need to see Fred. I tell Fred to page Anne and find out what they can do. Later, he says, Anne advises him to visit our local gastroenterologist. "What? Can't they help?" I tell Fred to call our GP; it's late, but maybe they are still there, and they will see him. He goes and gets some antibiotics. The diarrhea stops immediately.

Thursday, September 18, 2003

Paul comes to help with the work. We finish at 5 p.m. Fred comes to thank Paul. He has a hooded sweatshirt on and looks like a ghost.

Friday, September 19, 2003

On our way to Fox Chase, I ask Fred how he is. He replies, "I'm scared." I try to tell him that the diarrhea is unrelated and that we'll get to work on getting him back to feeling better and eating. He says, "Something has changed." Dr. Goldberg goes to get the PET scan results. I read to Fred as we wait. Waiting is unbearable. We have waited enough. Finally, he returns; the PET scan shows multiple other areas in the abdomen where something is happening and needs another CT scan to confirm. We take off for the CT scan. I sit with him and wait. After 45 minutes, they take him, and

I call Barbara and Jon to walk Tashie. Our electricity has been out since the hurricane. I go back to wait for Fred; he is walking in the hallway. We go back to the Imaging room to have them call Dr. Goldberg. Shortly after, he says the CT scan has confirmed multiple additional tumors are growing in his abdomen. Surgery is no longer an option. Only chemotherapy. He goes to get Dr. Cheng. We wait. Dr. Goldberg returns quickly and says that they will admit Fred right away. He doesn't look good, and they can stabilize him and maybe start chemotherapy in the hospital. This is overwhelming. I say, "I don't understand. Why does he have to go to the hospital?"

Admissions is ready for us. I call Mom. We don't really know what's going on. I tell Mom I'm scared. They whisk us to a room, and his nurse asks a list of questions: "Why are you here?" We say we're not sure. The admittance says dehydration. Dr. Cheng arrives and, after a few minutes, says, "Do you think you need to be here?" "No," we say, and I say, "I want him home," and Fred says he wants to go home. They stop the admission process. When Dr. Cheng returns to talk with us, I can tell he's in a hurry. But he sits. He says the tests confirm Fred's cancer has spread rapidly. August 20: a CT scan shows one spot on the lung. September 20: Another CT scan shows multiple additional spots in the abdomen. They have never seen it spread so fast. Now there is no hope for a cure. He has a few to many months left. They are hoping that chemotherapy will stop the disease and extend his life by a few to many months, but not years. He can decide not to have treatment; that's his choice. "You mean I can stay home and die?" "Yes," says Dr. Cheng. There is the possibility of a miracle—that the cancer will just go away. We decide on chemotherapy, which will begin on Monday. I cry in the car again while driving home, and Fred nods off.

We are not on the Road Back any longer.

Saturday, September 20, 2003

We can hardly breathe. I had a migraine last night, and I'm completely exhausted. I go out in the morning to the pool. It doesn't help. We live again in an altered state.

Sunday, September 21, 2003

Eileen calls. She will be Fred's nurse. We discuss his drugs, and I tell her to check on the steroids. She will start fluids and draw blood.

Monday, September 22, 2003: The last day of summer.

And the second round of chemotherapy begins. Mom takes Fred to the hospital. I get to the infusion room around 3 p.m. He is done. Eileen is demonstrating how to detach the portable infusion pack. We both practice, get supplies, and more prescriptions. He is already nauseous. On the way home, he says, "They'll have to do more than this to do me in!" I say, "Good, we need you to keep fighting." I remember him saying that after about three days of chemotherapy and radiation last year. He is sick all night; he tries to get to the bathroom in time every hour.

Tuesday, September 23, 2003

I wonder about Fred's daughter. I'm not sure she's called recently, and I'm not sure I should bother asking. Did she hear me? Should I call again or send a card?

Sunday, September 28, 2003

Mom stays over. Jon and Barbara come over to help finish the labeling. We set up production again, and Fred comes out to say it's lonely in the house.

I feel much better with everyone around. They say they want us to know we are not alone.

Friday, October 3, 2003

Fred disconnects his portable infusion pump. He looks forward to this activity. It is a constant reminder of the battle. He struggles to maintain some dignity and find some peace with the day. It is easier without the pump attached. The cancer takes away your strength, slowly sapping it away. It is easy to see that people will just diminish, getting weaker until they are unable to fight any longer.

Monday, October 6, 2003

Fred told me last night that he wants to get some saline and a Procrit shot. He is going to the hospital alone; I will man the harvest. I call the nurse and Dr. Cheng and leave messages saying he is at the hospital and what he wants. I hope they get the messages.

He comes home after noon. They were ready for him this time. He feels better than last week.

Tuesday, October 7, 2003

Fred's chemotherapy regimen is: Week 1–three drugs; weeks 2 and 3–one drug if not so sick; then repeat. We're bracing for next week with the three drugs. A friend brought us some marijuana to help with nausea. He is so weary; it's an effort to get through the day.

He is getting very quiet. Yesterday, I was away during the day; he said he was scared all day, scared of what's to come.

I have come to a place that knows

There must be hope.

No other way to continue.

There are lots of examples;

those with shortened futures;

who live anyway.

"Ludicrous," he says.

Wednesday, October 8, 2003

Cape Cod boy.

Sweet child of the sand and sea,

Your parents' gifts.

A stoic Finn, acting tough,

Hard as steel,

And gentle as the mist.

The beauty you see in the sunrise,

Every animal a treasure of life,

Connections with nature

Aloof, demanding, and difficult you seem

To those who know only

The passing interchange.

As the surfs are crashing,

The dunes are shifting,

The smell of the sea is blowing through the brain,

You are.

10/07/89

Happy anniversary!

Thursday, October 9, 2003

Sleep evades us. Fred can sleep for about 4 hours at a time. The chemotherapy drugs give him wild dreams. They also make his intestinal system quick. He stays close to home, close to the bathroom.

Saturday, October 18, 2003: Champagne Day

Fred sat out in the courtyard with sunglasses and a baseball cap. I was busy in the salesroom; he got very cold and finally went inside. Hypothermia was the diagnosis that night.

He has never admitted to being afraid.

Sunday, October 19, 2003

His hernias and varicose veins in his legs were hurting all night and all day today. He can barely stand. The thought of chemotherapy starting again tomorrow is making him sick. Last week, his doctors finally learned from us that he has constant diarrhea. My mother went to the hospital for an infusion on Monday, so I could keep working here. She asked his nurse, "What are you going to do about the diarrhea?" "What?" the nurse inquired before summoning his doctor. Dr. Cheng arrived and asked Fred how many times a day he had diarrhea. "About ten," says Fred. Dr. Chang says, "How long has this been going on?" "Since the start of chemotherapy," says Fred.

OH! So they have given him a week off and some prescription drugs that had to be ordered. On Saturday, I discovered that it could be an antibiotic. Things are getting very mixed up. Is this what happens to the patients? There seems to be less attention. The ball is being passed to the GP; there is too much of an opening for something to get missed. They are not listening to me. Why?

Tuesday, October 28, 2003

We call Deedee, our local nurse, to ask for an injection shot demo. His arms are all bruised, and one is bleeding. His blood is thinner. She shows how to do it.

Wednesday, October 29, 2003

We meet with Dr. Cheng. Fred is recuperating from blood clots and painful varicose veins. His weight is stable, but he needs to put 5 pounds back on – our own barometer. Fred asks about what's next. We learn they want to do a 4-month chemotherapy course with some breaks. A CT scan in three weeks will tell if this is keeping the cancer in check. They hope it's in check or reduced; we hope it's gone. "And then what?" Fred asks. "More chemotherapy," Dr. Cheng replies. "Am I going to live? Dr. Cheng replies slowly, "Yes," and mentions the chemotherapy being toxic and affecting his quality of life. I'm still hoping for a miracle.

I look Dr. Cheng in the eyes and say, "I know Fred will make it. I am doing everything I can think of to help him, and we want to know about everything that can help." He says that a positive attitude is good; it makes a difference. I ask him about his research and other research. I checked out his bio and tried to find research on the internet, but I didn't get much. I ask, "Are there a lot of other places working on esophageal cancer?" "Just pockets," he replies. I ask about sonar; he says, "There's not much on that, and the heat level isn't enough to break the cell's bonds. I talk about dolphins and say that we are going to go swimming with them when Fred can take a break. He says there is a new antibody effective against colon cancer that may be helpful. It is the only thing he thinks might work. But insurance won't cover it, and it costs $20,000. He says that maybe they could petition to get it, and I tell him I used to work in medical research at Penn and would volunteer to help in his lab.

Living with Death

Our next phase.

Sunday, November 2, 2003

Maybe we can escape to the beach this day—our first respite since the spring. Fred decides he doesn't want to go. He's worried about what the next CT scan will show.

I ask, "But wouldn't you enjoy seeing the beach?" "No," he says. "It's too late."

What can I do to make his day a little happier?

"So it was programmed in my genes that I would get cancer," he says.

I tell him I am so sorry that he is going through this. I wish every moment that it would go away. Lame, I am lame and unable to say anything of consequence.

Isn't there a way for him to still enjoy what life he has?

Monday, November 10, 2003

We'll go to Fox Chase today. At 6 a.m., Fred was vomiting in the bathroom, the spinach he said as I looked in the bowl, nerves I thought to myself. Did you take some anti-nausea stuff? Yes, the ashen face replied.

His hemoglobin was 12.6, never seen it that good in the last 14 months. Ten more pounds off the scale. How can this be? He's not drinking or eating very much, is afraid to have diarrhea, and is tired and weak. Is this a gradual decline? Hard to know where we're at. I talk about the visiting nurse- can't get it sorted out. They give him 2000 ml of saline. Someone finally looked at his mouth- yep, he's dehydrated!

Tomorrow the visiting infusion nurse is coming to add to my assignments.

I search the clinical trials.gov site for anything. Have lots to ask Cheng about.

The daughter and family are finally coming to visit on November 22.

Sister Nancy says she is also coming in early December...to pay her last respects.

I have to keep going. It feels like I am losing the battle of keeping it together. I am useless.

Denial, some are still in denial.

Last week the neighbor Real estate salesperson left her card in the door. Fred gets it and calls her. She says she heard he was ill, small talk; then she says she heard the vineyard was for sale. He says, "No, of course we will keep you in mind." The sharks and vultures are circling.

The drugs, I know the names; I can see them on the drip bags and big syringes: Cisplatin, 5FU, Epirubicin- the red bomb.

God, You have made a mistake. You can fix this; please fix this now.

Friday, November 14, 2003

The week seemed easier; we finally got the infusion nurse to come out with extra fluids on Thursday. She added acidophilus to help rebuild the good flora in the intestine. The diarrhea has subsided in the last few days.

Fred just told me he's feeling bad; the diarrhea started again last night, and he doesn't feel well. He wants to know about chemotherapy on Monday; Dr. Cheng told him maybe not next week. There's a CT scan on Monday. "Too bad," says Fred.

I'm feeling desperate. The noose is tightening, am I imagining it? We have never gotten good news. Please.

Monday, November 17, 2003

5 a.m.: we're up. Fred is unsteady and falls at the bottom of the stairs. He has been outside working this weekend. I give him a hug, and he says, "Is that before my execution?" There's a CT scan today with Dr. Cheng. We will know our fate. I am prepared for the worst. Fred is talkative on the way to the hospital. It feels like a nice morning with no foreboding. He says he figures the chemotherapy helped him before, which means there is a good chance it will help him again. I say only yes and work hard to chase the other possibilities from my brain. I drop him off and go swimming. I continue to practice looking down; I don't want any eye contact, and I don't want anyone to know my pain.

Noon: Elation, pure joy. The CT scan showed improvement, and the chemotherapy is working well. Finally, some good news. I call Mom on the way home. There are many calls to make to share the good news, and thanks for the prayers. Fred talks about his mother's sister, Bonnie, having some rare cancer and living with it for a long time, and his cousin, Carl, having brain cancer and living with it. He says he has been thinking that maybe his genes are predisposed to cancer but also carry the capability to live beyond it. I think about the fire coral in the sea—so toxic, yet the plant grows close to the anti-toxin. He asks, "Why do so many die from cancer?" I say, "They can't endure the treatment; they just give up." It's hard to do what he is doing to live. I say, "You are lucky to be alive." "Yes, maybe so." He says. He talks about getting good news when it was most important—after chemotherapy and radiation—that it worked well, and they thought he would keep some of his stomach. After surgery, he made it and kept over half his stomach. Later, with his Pyloric valve, it finally worked. And now, the chemotherapy is working and seemingly well. He says this will probably add several years to his life. And maybe more, if we can just keep going.

In the evening, Fred says this will take some getting used to. He has worried for the past year, but now it is different.

Tuesday, November 18, 2003

The visiting nurse has to wait for Fred to return. It's the first time he's been out in weeks. He went to get new jeans.

Wednesday, November 19, 2003

    Walking in the clouds,

    Sun flowing all around,

    Bathed in light and love,

    Snug, safe, and secure,

    There is hope.

    How quickly the change,

    Prepared for the worst,

    Maybe for the first

    Light steps, eye contact,

    Fun is around the corner.

Friday, November 21, 2003

The infusion pump is disconnected, meaning freedom for Fred. He gets a break next week—they encourage participation in "life events." The holidays qualify. I keep him eating.

Thanksgiving, 2003

A quiet beginning. Paul, Dad, Mom, and Izzy stop by on their way to Kathy's. Paul is finishing the grout at the edge of the beautiful stone walkways he constructed for us. Then we caravan to Kathy's. I have the makings of a champagne tasting. Everyone is involved and enjoys the opportunity. We wait for hours for dinner, laughing at the cooks. Finally, we are all seated and having a chatty dinner. Dad says a blessing. Mom is weakened by her car accident earlier in the week. She got rear-ended by an SUV that never slowed down. She was out cold for over an hour in the emergency room. I am worried about her.

Fred says he will be morose again in December—nothing personal. I say, "I know," and I only hope to help make it a little easier for him. "You must continue," I say. "Yes," he says. "I am sorry it is so hard."

Monday, December 1, 2003

The infusion room is not so crowded today. The blood lab only drew one tube, so we'll wait an hour for another lab test. His labs are OK. J&J has withdrawn

Procrit for chemotherapy patients because of increased blood clots. Fred has stopped taking the shots. His hemoglobin is 12.6; we now consider that normal for him. The pharmacy nurse says that chemotherapy patients frequently get blood clots anyway.

The Red bomb, epirubicin, goes mainline into the port artery. The nurse tells us it can burn a hole in muscle or veins. Fred is scared of this drug. It makes him sick. We are expecting a bad reaction in the next 36 hours.

Wednesday, December 3, 2003

We never expected this bad of a trip. Constant diarrhea. Since 7 a.m., he's been throwing up gross, discolored bile. He hasn't eaten in 48 hours. He has "pacing, moving leg syndrome." The extra fluids yesterday aren't making a difference. Rush to the pharmacy for some Zofran and more Sandistatin. The Zofran is working; he's sipping some Gatorade. At 9 p.m., he says he'll eat something. "What would you like?" "Coleslaw." "Coleslaw? "How about soft foods like mashed potatoes or eggs?" "No, I want coleslaw." "But don't you think you should start slow and easy?" "Whatever," whatever that means.

I make French toast: white bread soaked in egg and milk with a little butter and syrup. "What's that?" "French toast." He eats slowly and hands me the tray. "How did that go?"

"I'm full, it doesn't feel good, so I think I'll get rid of it." He walks out the front door and starts puking. "That feels better." I guess I should have just given him the coleslaw.

He falls asleep in the La-Z-Boy. He's more awake and feisty on Thursday.

The patient from hell is back.

Thursday, December 4, 2003

Little things, all day, "Did you do this? When are you going to do that? Run, run. What were you doing in the kitchen so long?" Minutes seem like hours to him. He talks a lot. I go to another winery to pick up some wine boxes, meet a carpenter about a custom railing and prepare a special order for pickup at 5 p.m. I check in at the house and discover the mad repairman has been working in the dining room again. Paint chips and plaster dust are scattered everywhere. The mad repairman doesn't cover anything up or clean up. Tracks from the dining room scatter the dust and paint chips around the downstairs. The trowels are in the sink; he used the wrong trowel again, not the serrated one. Uneven gobs of joint compound are smeared around the wall. The drill is lying on the bare fine dining room table. The vacuum is covered in dust. The antique oriental serves as a drop cloth. I shake my head and say it isn't worth getting upset about. "I'll clean it up."

8 p.m.: "Survivor," which we both enjoy watching for its insightful commentary on social behavior. This group is a bunch of liars. The women are so gullible they keep believing whatever the men tell them. It's four women and two men, and the four women can't figure out they are in the driver's seat. I fall asleep on the floor and can't seem to stay up past 9 p.m.

11 p.m.: I finally go upstairs; Fred has napped and is now awake.

1 a.m.: He comes up to get something, and I ask him to turn the volume down on the TV.

3 a.m.: Fred asks where the syringes are. I reply, "Wait until morning, and I'll disconnect your pump." "Where are the syringes?" He asks again, ignoring my suggestion. I reply, "They're hanging up in the closet in a blue bag." He's already gone before I've finished speaking. After 2 minutes, I get up to help; he may take a shortcut that isn't safe. I flush the two lines after explaining again why we have to flush. Saline and heparin. As I go upstairs, he asks, "Where are you going?"

"To try to get some sleep. I'll disconnect your port butterflies in the morning. You'll just have to wait."

4 a.m.: "Where is the letter I was working on?"

5 a.m.: He calls upstairs, something about a telephone number he can't read. "Bring it up here."

All the lights go on. "It's *82."

"Oh, I never would have guessed," he says, walking away.

"You're going to call Miguel now?"

"Yes."

"But it's 5 a.m."

"Yes."

It's quiet for a few minutes.

At 5:15, I give up and get up.

I have to start early anyway, with the storm coming.

7 a.m.: I leave for printers, the pool, and groceries.

10 a.m.: I arrive back. He gets into the car as I start to unload it; he has to go to the hardware store. He can't wait; I grab a bag before he pulls away. The mad repairman is back—more of the same as yesterday. I quickly vacuum the big stuff and roll up the oriental rug part way, clearing all the chairs from one side of the room. Dave's waiting for more champagne disgorgement and custom labeling.

3 p.m.: I head over to the house to check on Fred. There are only a few inches of snow. His car is missing. Inside, the mad repairman has made a really big mess. The sander has had a field day. Everything in the room is covered with plaster dust; one of the chairs acts as a ladder, and the work area has been expanded. The dust has spilled over into the kitchen and the living room. Patience is nowhere to be found. Now I'm tracking it all over the house. I try to clear a path.

4 p.m.: The mad repairman returns and says he had an accident. I say, "I told you not to go out." He needed plastic to cover up the dining room. I say, "Now, you're going to cover things up? Why didn't you yesterday?" Anyway, as I have already said, patience has already left the building.

Sister Kathy to the rescue—we need to get patience back. We talk about patterns in our lives, patterns gotten from our parents. I say that nothing is important—all those little things that seemed important aren't. Changing one's behavior is hard. We all start from different places. I think about things I've learned over the last decade:

Look for patterns in my behavior and the relationship.

Is there evidence that change has taken place?

Don't assume.

Expectations frequently lead to disappointment.

Move forward.

And most important: get more of what I need from myself.

Later, I apologize to Fred that I haven't been patient.

He says, "It started yesterday."

"Yes, my patience has been low since yesterday."

"What is the reason?"

"I don't know, nothing in particular."

We start over.

I cook the venison chops from Marsha's husband, Chuck. He has just undergone treatment for prostate and bladder cancer. He's all clear, and his lymph nodes are negative. Cancer: an epidemic.

I realize the groceries are still in Fred's car. I go out to get them, and the car is missing—it's up at the mechanic's already. Melting ice pops will await us on Monday.

Sunday, December 6, 2003

Twelve inches of snow—the first winter snowstorm. Last year, a winter snowstorm hit on the same date. Curious. Everything is closed. I work in the winery on special orders.

Amazingly, the electricity is still on. We dig ourselves out.

Wednesday, December 9, 2003

Fred is doing better and eating better. He says he visited the GP's office today for an allergy shot. The nurse came out to the car to give him his shot. They apparently do this a lot in flu season, especially this year, and especially for Fred.

Thursday night, Bonnie calls. Doug got us a Christmas tree. I immerse it in water on the front porch when he brings it up. Fred says he doesn't want it. Later, he says he's not going to help put it up. "I know," I say and pat him.

Saturday, December 13, 2003

We're ready in the winery; where are the customers? The room is nicely decorated with more gifts and special items. I finish putting up bows, greens, and wreaths outside. We go for an understated, elegant look. Our wine is similar. Another storm is on the way, with ice this time. I do another state store champagne tasting; it's too busy, so I change the time to 5 p.m. in King of Prussia. Good store, poor access. Pennsylvania regulates all alcoholic beverage sales through its

350+ stores. They ordered 20 cases of our champagne at 50% off our retail price, one per store in Eastern Pennsylvania, and we had to go to each store to put it on the shelf, buy a bottle, and give in-store tastings. That's the big support from the state. We sold a few bottles and provided the most in-store tastings to date. It's too late for Fred to eat when I'm done. I stop for pizza, eat it in the car, and finish with a glass of champagne—little things to feel like I'm still among the living.

Tuesday, December 16, 2003

He was up all night, banging on the walls, with the TV and lights on to keep him company—maybe to keep the thoughts of terror at bay. I notice his feet are swollen. This starts a spiral in my head about what could be the cause. I examine his legs; they are basically not swollen above the ankles.

"Is this good?" I offer the heating pad and suggest he put his feet up. I will try to put it out of my mind until tomorrow when we see Dr. Cheng.

Wednesday, December 17, 2003

Fred doesn't want to go to the hospital. He asks, "Why can't we just talk on the phone?" I know this drill. "He needs to see you on a regular basis while you're on chemotherapy." "But I was just at the hospital." "I know, but your feet are swollen—we need to check that." Silence. I tell him that this is the first time things are stable with him since starting chemotherapy this fall. I recount all the things that have been wrong.

"Everything is fine; you look good—much better than the last time I saw you," says Dr. Cheng. Things are stabilized. Fred asks about his hernia again and when he can get it fixed. We press for an answer. Again, we are told to go to a general surgeon; the cancer doctors don't do this surgery. And then he says the surgeons don't like to do surgery on cancer patients. "Why?" I ask. He replies, "I don't know, really. Perhaps they consider the potential benefit and the discomfort of the surgery for someone in your situation." What does he mean? I feel a little hole opening in my armor. The box of doubts is open again. At night, I check to see if Fred is still breathing.

Thursday, December 18, 2003

More disgorgement is underway as we prepare for the weekend and, hopefully, a flurry of sales at the winery. With more baskets and decorations, I finally put the lights on our house tree. Fred says it's nice.

It's Christmas time, and we live in total clutter and debris. He calls me a moron; maybe I am. And why does he have to have the TV on 24 hours a day? All night I have to hear the TV and have the lights on. He asks, "Can you hear the TV?" I reply, "Yes, I hear everything, and the light keeps me awake." He then asks, "Do you have the door closed?" I sigh and go to bed.

Friday, December 19, 2003

We finish decorating our tree without tinsel. Fred has cleaned up the house while I'm out doing errands. He apologizes for calling me a moron. I apologize for getting mad; I was overly tired. I give him warm, wet paper towels and tell him to clean off his fingers and the area under his nose covered in dried blood. I ask him, "Is your nose bleeding anymore?" He replies, "It bled for 20 minutes yesterday; I thought it wouldn't stop." Now, what to do?

Saturday, December 20, 2003

Fred says his feet are swollen and don't fit in any shoes. And his nose keeps bleeding. Stop picking at your nose. I have to get the crud out. I clean up the trail of bloody tissues and get a clean trash bag. He's upset I'm not around more and sulks like a baby. He's right; I haven't been a good nurse lately.

At night, he says the latest "roofer" recommended sending his son to pick up the trailer and ladder they left four weeks ago when they said they would replace the stone house roof. It will get new shakes someday. Fred tells his son that is bullshit; they are not here doing the job. The son is apparently surprised and says he will get his father to call us tonight. We don't expect to hear from them again. Good for Fred.

Sunday, December 21, 2003

I try to return to the house more often and check

on him. Mom and Kathy come for a holiday visit. We hang out in the winery. Fred gets a little visit, but he clearly doesn't want company. When I ask if I can get him anything, he says, "Go away."

Monday, December 22, 2003

Fred is upset because a customer came while I was out and had to hobble over to the winery. His feet are still swollen. "OK, sit down and put your feet up." He's so stubborn; he hasn't been doing that. I don't feel sorry for him today.

Tuesday, December 23, 2003

In the afternoon, he gets another nosebleed that won't stop. I check his feet and ankles and discover they are all red and blotchy. Now what? I call his nurse. She and Dr. Cheng are both already gone for the holiday. I leave a message for the backup nurse and call Mom. The nurse calls back, and we discuss the present symptoms. "What about the blood thinner?" "Maybe, but Lovenox is not supposed to need the monitoring that Heparin does." She talks to Dr.

Meropol. They want Fred to come in for blood work and wait to see the doctor if something is amiss. He says emphatically, "No, he won't go anywhere." I tell the nurse we'll discuss this, and I'll call back. I yell at him to put his feet up. He wouldn't do this for the past week, and now we're up against the holiday, and it's another crisis. He says he's just trying to survive.

He does put his feet up above his heart level. After two hours, his toes are much better. I say we'll decide tomorrow what to do. He doesn't want the blood thinner shot. I say, "OK."

I go to bed with visions of normalcy in my head.

Wednesday, December 24, 2003

I sleep in until 7 a.m. I have to get up, but I don't want to face the day. I ask, "How are you?" He replies, "Fine." I say, "Let me check your feet." A little tug, then he relents. There's not much improvement. I say, "In the last 12 hours, for how many hours have your feet been up?" "3-4," he says. I can't believe it. I say, "You need to do more. 50% of the time. What are we going to do about the Lovenox?" No answer. I continue, "We just can't stop taking it." He says, "It's been three months; isn't that enough?" I reply, "I don't know." He says, "First, Dr. Cheng said three months; last week, he said at least four months." I ask, "What about your nose bleeds?" Silence. He turns his back on me. He says, "I have to do something." I call Mom and ask her, "What should I do?" We discuss the options. She recommends going for the blood test; then, we will know if the level is OK. I say, "Alright, I'll go tell Fred we are going to the hospital." "I don't want to go," he yells. We have to know what's going on. We can't make a good decision. I tell him I'm sorry; I know it's hard for him. And having all of these ongoing symptoms must be annoying for him. I'm sure this is not life-threatening, but we can't ignore them. If we get it straightened out, he should start to feel better. I tell him, "Come on, get up; we're going." There's silence during the drive. I've left messages for the nurse stating that we're on our way and leave my cell phone number. I forgot to give him a Lovenox shot; will the tests be accurate? The nurse calls just as we get there and says they want us to come anyway.

We wait patiently. Finally, Dr. Meripol calls the lab

waiting room for Fred. Fred nudges me, and I answer the phone. "Hello, this is Janet, Fred's wife." He says, "The blood test shows everything is normal, including clotting levels and platelets." He asks about the timeline of events and whether we are on a treatment cycle now. We discuss going off the blood thinner. He agrees that it may make sense during the break. We know the risks: He could get another clot, which could go to his heart and cause him to die. I ask, "What about one shot a day instead of two?" "That is a compromise," says Dr. M. He agrees with that approach. He says, "Let them know how he is doing on Monday." I tell Fred, "We're out of here; I'll fill you in—in the car." He waits by the main entrance in his down booties, the only thing that fits his swollen feet and ankles.

Thursday, December 25, 2003

To survive,

The patient musters the energy of his ancestors,

Finns, Russian persecution,

Tough, enduring, strong constitutions

Surviving in the face of towering odds.

Facing the enemy

Time and time again

Never give up

Never give in.

Learn, evolve, finesse.

Decide a response

Stay the course

To the bitter end.

Like a Holocaust victim,

Never knowing if there will be a tomorrow.

I am the communicator,

The caregiver,

The assistant.

I must know how it is,

I must be ever vigilant.

Seek out the path

Seek out the difference makers

Support the effort

Keep the path clear,

The seemingly insignificant yet annoying side effects.

Each body has its own style of dealing with the stress.

Look for hope.

Find hope

Provide hope.

We must go on

For that is what life is.

Merry Christmas, 2003

Sunday, December 28, 2003

Fred has been having very tough days. I can see his mental struggle. He must face his mortality every minute. When I check on him in the middle of the night, he is sitting awake in the La-Z-Boy. He catnaps. I think he hopes for sleep to escape the dread of being awake, but sleep mostly escapes him. His lips are set in resolve, the stoic Finn. Please, can I find something to give him a smile?

Monday, December 29, 2003

Now I am writing just to talk to someone. Initially, my mother encouraged me to keep a journal because "people will want to read it," she said.

It has been a godsend for me to recount each day's events; it's calming and lets me go on.

I can barely write that Fred is diminishing before my eyes. Slowly, his speech falters, his memory is bare, engagement belongs in the eyes of the beholder, the chemotherapy is minimizing his being, he wants only to survive, and I want him to hold on. We will get the antibody C225. I see the letter and numbers getting bigger in my thoughts. Whispers return now and then: "…died after a long battle with cancer." I fight to focus on the possibilities–that there are possibilities. I fight to believe and have hope. He depends on me to do the best thing. I hope I have not let him down.

Please, God, we need the other miracle now.

Tuesday, December 30, 2003

I pay all the bills and just discovered our medical insurance went up 50%!

Wednesday, December 31, 2003

New Year's Eve. We have survived another year, and the winery has had significant growth. We have created a niche in the local wine market but took the long, slow, and very hard route—organic growth. We focus on quality and the experience of visiting us. Next year is our tenth year in business. They say that's where the rubber meets the road in small business.

Fred is so tired he can barely get up. Yesterday I had to pull him up from the couch. I finally reached the home health pharmacy and got him a lower chest support wrap to help with the stomach hernia. It sticks out and looks like he has an alien about to pop out. Also, they had the wedge pillows that many have suggested. The nurse recommended trying a 7-inch one for starters. When Fred saw it, he considered using it to elevate his feet. The ankles are still swollen but holding. Improvement is slight and occurs weekly.

Later, we hold hands, and Fred thanks me for all I have done. I say, "That's nothing, and we have more to do next year!" I go to bed at 10:30 and have already forgotten about the celebration. At midnight, some local fireworks and hoorahs wake me up. Tashie barely stirs; I touch her and give thanks again.

New Year's Day, 2004

Fred says he is so tired and weak. His quality of life is not good. What if the next CT scan shows no improvement? I feel the ancestors are with me now; I feel strong again. I say with authority and assurance that there is no way there won't be an improvement. After six weeks, there was a significant improvement; after two more chemotherapy cycles, there will be much more. The hope is that all the spots get resolved. Then we will get the antibody C225 to prevent any more tumors from growing. He is thinking. I hope I have been convincing. I made an appointment at the University of Pennsylvania with a surgeon who is also a surgical oncologist. I tell Fred he will probably have to wait for the hernia surgery until after the chemotherapy cycles. He asks, "What is the schedule?" I talk about the three more cycles and say they shouldn't be as bad as these last three. He had a blood clot, endless diarrhea, dehydration, and nausea. I say, "Let's review what we should do next week to deal with those symptoms. I feel I have not done a good job of remembering and thinking ahead about what to do for my New Year's resolution." He falls silent—enough of that. A little later, I get the Lovenox shot, and there is no other box—how can this be? We were on one shot a day and should have another box of 10 shots. I look everywhere. Of course, something always happens on holidays. We have to wait until tomorrow. What if he gets a new clot today, and it goes to his heart? I am beside myself.

We had semi-planned to go away overnight to the shore—an idea since we learned of the disease's spread. Kathy and Rick offered their condo at Rehoboth Beach, Delaware. We planned to go today. The thought of getting everything together for an overnight trip feels monumental. Fred can't sleep in a bed. He would be sitting up half the night. Yesterday, I suggested a day trip. This morning, Fred said he didn't want to go. Relief. It probably would be good to get away, but we need a driver at least. I'm tired from the year and usually look forward to the holidays to recharge. Today I will work on that.

Friday, January 2, 2004

Fred is anxious and says he's scared of what's to come. I try to comfort him, but I don't have anything really good to say. Monday is back to "House of Horrors."

At night, we discuss money, equipment needs, and capital projects like solar. He is upset and challenges me to get more work. I don't like the approach, so I push back. We each give our views of our finances. The truth is, it's precarious. I am optimistic; he is pessimistic. It feels like old times.

Saturday, January 3, 2004

We have always hoped to add solar electricity to our buildings. We have been researching a grant. The consultant and installer meet us, answer questions, and discuss battery backup and a split system with trackers and a unit on the roof. It's the first time in months that Fred really engages in the discussion. He is fully in the present. It's so nice to see. This is a good project for the next six months to keep him involved.

Sunday, January 4, 2004

He got reflux at dinner last night and had it all night. At 4 a.m., he comes up to bed for a few hours. In the morning, he says he's scared. "About tomorrow?" I ask. He nods yes. I say, "It won't be as bad. Take some Ativan today." He replies, "OK."

I am Abenaki,

And German, French, and English.

Of the Wabanaki's of Quebec.

He is Finn,

Carramaki, Of the little Hill,

And now of Cape Cod.

We have strong ancestors,

Of the sea and the land.

It is in our blood,

I feel their influence,

Protect the animals of the sea and the land.

It is our duty and privilege to know them.

Surround us with your light.

Protect us from the sounds of silence.

I am terrified. Tomorrow begins the siege again.

Monday, January 5, 2004

5 a.m.: Poor Fred struggled all day yesterday and could barely move. I held his hands, kissed him warmly, and tried comforting him. He's worried about the future. He had reflux all night and some congestion; I'll have to ask about that. It's back to Fox Chase, the House of Horrors, today. Epirubicin is a scary, very potent drug. The siege begins again for the next three weeks. There is nothing to look forward to except the hope of a good CT scan in three weeks. How would you fare?

Tuesday, January 6, 2004

The first thing Fred said when I came downstairs this morning was that Tug McGraw, a former Phillies pitcher, had died of brain cancer.

Yesterday was better than the last three cycles. Fred ate dinner and got some sleep. Anne came to see us in the infusion room. She thinks the swollen feet and ankles may be a protein problem - he needs to eat better. I haven't been watching as closely; I need to work on it. He promised to eat more. She said the basketball-looking stomach might be fluids due to a protein problem or the cancer. It makes little fluid sacs in that area. My alarms went off. I didn't want to ask any more questions, but I'm thinking, "Isn't the chemotherapy killing the cancer cells? Or is this basketball-looking area a mass of tumors?" Poor Fred, he must be very scared. I have to keep going and keep thinking there is hope. Two weeks till the CT scan. I feel my nerves convulsing; that will be the underlying feeling for the next two weeks.

The nurse comes to connect his other port. He doesn't want any infusions today. OK, just let the nurse access your other port. Try to eat.

Wednesday, January 7, 2004

I'm looking at the saline bag and realize that in my hurry to get the visiting nurse in and out quickly, I forgot to have her hook up the bag. I call their office; they are fantastic; someone always answers the phone, and they can always help over the phone. God bless them. She talks me through connecting the tubing, and I manage to connect it without losing the saline. I set Fred up with the IV machine and get the walkie-talkies. I'll be in the winery disgorging champagne again with Dave. I say, "Let's check them—I'll go in the other room—can you hear me now?" The static beep sound. I go back into the living room and tell him to try again. His fingers are slow, and they release the button. He tries again to hold the button down. He does. "I say, there, we can reach each other! I'll check in on you at lunch; keep your feet up!"

At night, he knocks over the cranberry juice all over the standing tray as I serve him dinner. He says, "I'm sorry," as I leave the room. I say, "No problem," and hope I am not showing any adverse body language. I think of the Fox Chase Cancer Center sign: "We are committed to treating with dignity and reducing the burden of human cancer." I am committed to treating Fred with dignity and preserving his dignity.

Thursday, January 8, 2004

Morning chores, "Want to check my feet?" he says with interest. I pull his down booties off that he's been wearing for six weeks–definite improvement! I say, "Good job!" He smiles. I put lotion on his feet and suggest a shower when we unhook his fanny pack tomorrow. "I washed the booties," he says. I smile, kiss him all over his face, and rub his head. I keep a smile on at all times.

I get his lunch at noon and then leave for the pool and meetings downtown. I am down when I leave the house. I'm still worried about what Anne said about the stomach area. Can that be a tumor or tumors that are growing? It had not entered my mind before Anne's comment. On my way home, I reach Mom. She felt his distended stomach; did she think it was a tumor? "No," she says. I ask, "Can I still have hope?" She says, "Yes, you must always have hope. If Fred wants to live, he will live. Do you have any other information?" I reply, "No, till the next CT scan." So we wait, and I have hope. I am right to have hope. I need to just keep going. God bless Mom.

At night, I tell Fred to wake me up when he wants

to disconnect his pump. I ask, "5 a.m.?" He replies, "Yes, 5 a.m. is great if you can wait until then." I tuck him in the La-Z-Boy, turn the TV on, and turn the lights out.

Friday, January 9, 2004

I'm up at 6:30, and he's already disconnected the pump. I ask, "Did you flush the ports?" He replies, "Yes." I ask again, "Did you take out the port needles?" He replies, "Yes." The box of supplies is open on the floor. Later, he says we are short on heparin. I ask, "Did you flush with heparin?" He replies, "Yes." Later he says he could only find one heparin; he can't remember where the other supplies are. I ask, "Which port did you flush with heparin?" He replies, "Pump one." I say, "OK. Next time, wake me up." Later, I think I should lay everything out the night before.

I encourage him to eat more and give him a morning boost. Then I'm off to Harrisburg to meet with a senator about support for our solar project. I then go to the Secretary of Agriculture's reception and bring Fred home a piece of cake. At night, he eats dinner and then gets milk and cake. Within ten minutes, he's in the bathroom throwing up. He says, "Don't talk to me again about eating!" This is familiar; I focus on getting him to eat more, and he seemingly goes along until he throws up, then tells me to butt out. Nothing is perfect.

Saturday, January 10, 2004

I give him warm cloths to wipe the blood off his hands and nose, but he still struggles with nose bleeds. I'm careful not to mention food. Later, I suggest he count calories to help him monitor his intake. "No, there is no need." I probably should do this.

Sunday, January 11, 2004

I'm trying not to think about the week. I have an underlying feeling of uneasiness. I have been fantasizing about the future—a leap from the present to the future, where there is happiness. I cry on the way back from the pool; I have to get out and get away; I have a moment of total terror. The floor is slipping away.

Monday, January 12, 2004

I'm up early, preparing us for the House of Horrors. Fred asks if I am going with him. I reply, "Yes, how could you go alone?" He's still in his down booties, with his big feet and ankles. I drop him off at the main entrance and go park. I swim when I get home and stay with him at the hospital. I stand up in the waiting room with a stiff back. I watch him walk slowly into the blood draw room; he staggers slightly. Some faces are familiar. Many people chat away, seemingly oblivious to the many life-and-death struggles in the room. People say, "Excuse me," to Fred, who is half out of it, so he will move his legs, and they can get by. I try to screen him from these people and look at them like, "Can't you see he can hardly move?" His blood work is OK; his hemoglobin is at 11, and he's holding. We get out in 2 hours, a record, and have burgers and fries on the way. We get home before noon.

I work in the winery and leave for the pool late afternoon. I cry, going to and from the car. I am overwhelmingly sad and keep fantasizing about the future, similar to when I was young. Somehow things will be all right; after all, I will live.

Tuesday, January 13, 2004

I can't stop crying. I am so scared. I keep thinking about his growing stomach—are they bunches of tumors? He is so diminished, with thin, bony, and hanging skin. He has been awake all night due to reflux. He was puking and gagging last night due to reflux. My future will surely be bright. I must stay 100% focused on the here and now to help him. Am I making a difference? I need to try harder. I bury myself in work at the winery and just check on him several times.

At 4 p.m., I get over to the house, and he is talking to the local doctor's office about getting an allergy shot. I say, "Give me a minute to change, and I'll drive you." We have to wait for the nurse—usually, they give Fred priority, but it's not the regular nurse today. Then we go to the pharmacy to pick up prescriptions. They're not ready, and Fred had only called in one of the three. The other two are too soon to fill. I tell Fred when I get back to the car. He says nothing. At home, he asks for prescriptions. I tell him again, and he gets upset and asks me, "Why didn't I tell him?" This is going nowhere; I look at the RXs and see we were at the doctor, and they could have called in a change if I knew. I have to do better. Now that it's almost 5 p.m., their office is closed. He tells me to call Fox Chase and says he needs the Ativan. So I start down that path, and FC proves again why they are so good: the patient comes first, they can handle my request, and they can get a new prescription called in before our pharmacy closes. I stop by Jon and Barbara's on the way and start crying furiously. I can't seem to stop. I'm afraid.

Wednesday, January 14, 2004

He's not eating; munching on cole slaw and chicken fingers at night. This behavior reminds me of his eating poorly after surgery. I feel like a mess, crying every time I leave the house. I feel like I am losing the battle. Is there hope? I try to reach Mom, my hope queen, but she doesn't answer.

Thursday, January 15, 2004

I get up early, organize my day, and force myself to get busy. I'm off to see our state representative about our solar project. The only thing new on the horizon is an anchor for Fred. That evening he is holding his head, saying, "What am I to do?" I try to be positive, but keeping Fred's two realities separate is hard. Reality 1 is that Fred will make it, and I speak only of this reality. Then there's reality 2–the doubt reality. And reality 2 has been fed to me a lot lately. What about his growing stomach area? I finally reach the hope queen–I am in the grocery store parking lot. I update her and say how scared I am. I ask, "Can you come visit?" "Yes," she says, thinking about how she will do that with her already overbooked schedule. I feel bad asking. She listens and says that maybe my imagination has run away with me. Maybe. "Patients who want to live do so, and Fred wants to live." We won't actually know what's going on until the CT scan on Monday. She asks about the albumin level, and we talk about getting that checked again. The doctors act on trends, not on a single test number. I will call and have them add a comprehensive blood test. She says, "Sometimes the nurses don't help; they don't always know what's really going on. Wait for the CT scan, then two days to see the doctor–that's the telling." I say, "Yes, we are waiting for the next telling." I cry again on the way home–*why do I keep doing that?*

Friday, January 16, 2004

I work until noon; then, I tell Fred we have to go to the hospital for his MUGA test. He says, "What? Can't I go next week?" I explain that we blew the test off over the holidays, and now they will keep asking and make us do it, so let's just get it done. And they can't do it on Monday when he goes for his infusion hookup. "What do you mean? I thought I was done with chemotherapy." I go through a few things, being careful not to mention the CT scan. At this point, I realize it's better for him and me not to tell him until the last minute. When we arrive at the Diagnostic Imaging department, I introduce him and give the receptionist his red card. She launches into her phone call reminder routine about the CT scan on Monday. She looks back and forth between us as she happily gets this off her list: "Your CT scan is scheduled for 8:30 on Monday; no food or drink after midnight, and do you have the drink?" I am ready to jump across the desk and strangle her, but I say, "We are here for a MUGA test; he doesn't know about any other tests," and I glare at her. She looks down and says, "Have a seat."

Five minutes later, Fred says he will need an anti-nausea pill. I have not brought the suitcase of drugs with me, so I ask the receptionist to please get a nurse who can get him something. She says they don't do that, and I should go to triage, and she proceeds to start telling me where triage is. I say, "I know where it is; please call Dr. Cheng." She glares back, dials a number, saying he doesn't answer, and hangs up the phone. I try again to get action, and she says, "You'll have to go to triage." The nurse comes out to get Fred, and I try to get her to get an anti-nausea pill, but there is no reaction. She says, "You can go to triage if you like; that's up to you." Fred decides to try it, and I say I will try to get him something. I try to hold my head up as the tears stream down my face as I walk to triage. Why am I crying? This feels so overwhelming—he just needs some anti-nausea medications. At triage, they are very sympathetic: "They shouldn't have made you come here." She pages Dr. Cheng, who calls right away and says to bring Fred back there after the test. She tells him twice that I am very upset. I'm not that upset and hope I have not made a mountain out of a molehill. It's often hard to know what is important and what is not. I hide in the ladies' room to get my composure and talk to myself. I can't help Fred if I am so upset, so I calm down.

Dr. Cheng decides not to wait and comes to the imaging area to talk with me. He has already talked to Fred. He motions me into the hall. My hackles stir, and I wonder if this is bad news. He says, "Fred is undernourished and not sleeping; he's very weak." I say, "Yes, and he had reflux all night long." He writes new prescriptions for a stronger sleep aid and an anti-nausea drug. We talk about the reflux and taking the medications every day. He says there will be no chemotherapy next week. I say, "But what about his stomach?" He makes that expression that he does and says, "Yes." I ask, "Is that a tumor growing?" He replies, "We don't know what's going on; the CT scan will tell us." He says he knows this is a very difficult time. I nod and ask, "In December, did you tell us the truth about the CT scan showing improvement?" He replies, "Yes." I ask, "Then is it reasonable to assume it's still improving?" He replies, "Yes, but that's what the CT scan will show." I ask, "And what about the C225-Erbitux? Can that help now?" He replies, "Possibly, it will be released in February, but your insurance will not cover it, and it's expensive—$10,000." "We'll have to find a way to get it," I say, thinking that the last three times I've asked about the antibody, he has said it would cost $20,000. Is he negotiating the price? "Thank you for seeing us, and have a good weekend," I say, trying to keep up a "together" image.

It seems like forever, and the nurse brings Fred out, saying he needs to get some more food in him and take care. They do a good job of recovering from a bad situation. I assist him in walking to the car. He wants to know what Cheng told me. I say, "Nothing earth-shattering, but you need to eat more." He asks, "Did he tell you that?" I reply, "Yes."

At night, I get my energy up to institute the new rules again: no eating after 8 p.m., more protein, and a nutritional drink per day. "I don't want to," he says. "I don't care; you need to do this," I say. He looks me in the eye. I think there is a little smile. Is he testing me to see if I am still engaged?

Sunday, January 18, 2004

I will not be downtrodden. That's easy for me to say because I will live. I draw energy from life; Fred must try. I tell him he doesn't know what will happen. And repeat that the drugs were recently helpful; they will be again. He has to work on eating better. I tell him, "Keep your feet up."

I didn't feel responsible for his poor nutrition when Dr. Cheng was talking. It's Fred's job to eat right, and I tell him so. I am doing all that I can do—or am I?

Fred says he doesn't want to go anywhere this week. I say, "OK, we'll reschedule everything," which is a royal nightmare, but truthfully, I have had enough of the hospital and people coughing near me for a while now.

Monday, January 19, 2004

It's a free day, so I work on the annual winery BATF reports. "What will I do?" That's the unanswerable question. The future will come. I will deal with it and go on. "There's no emotion left."

In the afternoon, I look out the kitchen window at a pair of red foxes making their way across the vineyard. Tashie must be asleep. The foxes like to come near our house in the middle of the night and make a shrieking, baying sound. There is no ignoring it, and Tashie matches them one for one with a ferocious bark until they move away.

Tuesday, January 20, 2004

Dave arrives, and we set up to start disgorging. We have to take advantage of the cooler weather. Dave asks a lot of questions about Fred. Last week, he just listened as I babbled along. He wants to know what the status is. Truthfully, I don't know. I relay the last week's happenings. We won't know until the CT scan. It's easy to let your imagination run away with you. The distended stomach is a concern, and Fred seems to be on a downward path. This chemotherapy is really taking it out of him. "And the weather is bad and cold," says Dave. "And it's hard to find hope sometimes," I say. He says, "Yes." Later, Dave tells me about a young woman at their church who, two years ago, was told she was terminal with some kind of cancer. Now there is no sign of it. I say, "Really? What kind was it, and how was she treated?" He's unsure of the type but thinks it's in the digestive area, and she got treatment and then said enough treatment, and now there is no sign of it! He has given me hope, and I believe that it can happen.

Wednesday, January 21, 2004

Fred goes for a walk up the vineyard hill and back. He's wiped out and feels awful when he returns. His legs looked swollen this morning, and I had to talk firmly about putting his feet up and nourishing his body better. He drank the nutritional drink in short order—no complaints. I tell him Dave's story about the young girl with no trace of cancer. He says, "Oh," nods, and meets my eyes.

Thursday, January 22, 2004

Last night, Tashie tortured me all night. She didn't sleep; she was hopping around the bed, whimpering at the critters outside, jumping around my head, up on the bed's headstand, her body tight as a drum. I could barely move her away; her strength is beyond her looks. There was no moving her off her watch. In the morning, she races out the door to check on the critter smells left behind. I check the back compost pile, and it looks like there was a deer party.

I call the hospital again and finally have Fred's appointments rescheduled. Monday is the CT scan.

Friday, January 23, 2004

Fred tells me I'm talking to myself more. "Oh," I say, thinking, *who else would want to listen to me?*

Is it the chemotherapy that has made him so weak? The questions just won't leave me any peace.

Thankfully, he gets a nap. When I walk into the room and see him sleeping, I continue my ritual of checking to see if his chest is moving.

The wind chill today is minus 10. I tell Tashie to spend only ten minutes at a time outside; after all, she has no shoes on.

At the Y, I donate $5 to the aquatics staff for the

Race for Life fundraiser. They give you a paper fish to decorate as you would like. The lifeguard looks at me funny when I say I want to buy a fish. "You're the first one," he says. That's a main theme in my life. As I swim, I start crying as I think about putting Fred's name on the fish. What will I say if they ask who he is? "You're supposed to put your name on the fish," says the lifeguard. But Fred's name needs to be there. I am crying as if I am telling someone about his disease. Ultimately, I hand the fish to another lifeguard, and no questions are asked.

But two little words are creeping into my thoughts: dying and terminal. And I am fleeing to a fantasy of my future when there is no cancer in my life and only light and happiness.

I drive to the store, realize I'm missing my purse, drive home, and then back again. I am mastering patience. At 10:30 p.m., I prepare to go to bed, and Fred says, "Can you stay up a little longer?" Yes, of course, and I hug him, kiss his sunken cheeks, and rub his head. I make tea and sit up for another hour. I tell him I'll make a bed downstairs to keep him company. He says he will keep me up all night.

Saturday, January 24, 2004

6° last night, with a dusting of snow and lots of wind. I've been fighting a cold for the last week and a half. And finally, I figured out that Fred has one too. That explains his mucus. I gave him decongestants yesterday, and last night he was better. That means extra time at the Y to spend in the steam room—what a luxury!

Before bedtime, Fred gets up to use the "outhouse" on the front porch. He stands in the living room and walks around in a circle. He looks in his pockets. I ask in a helping tone, "What are you looking for?" "Life," he says.

Sunday, January 25, 2004

We begin our morning routines: I say, "How are you? Did you get any sleep last night? Would you like coffee, tea, or bouillon this morning?" He replies, "Coffee." I say, "Later, are you ready for breakfast?" He says, "No, I'm not hungry." "You have to eat," I say. In a little while, I will say it again. I say, "OK. Farina, brown sugar, and a little milk—200 calories.

Pills. A nutritional drink?" He says, "No, don't talk to me about food." In a little while, he says, he's been thinking–there's a snowstorm tomorrow. I say, "Yes there is." He says, "I think I need to be in the hospital." I never expected this, but I am instantly relieved. We're not progressing, and I don't know what to do. I can hardly contain my relief and fight the urge to say, "Let's go." We talk a little, and I say, "Let's think about it. It is Sunday, so there will be work making it happen." I start doing some winery work, and finally, he says, "Call the hospital now."

And so I do. Fox Chase is not a regular hospital; they don't have an emergency room. We have to go to Jeannes Hospital's ER, and they will determine if he should be admitted. I start preparing things: the house, the dog, the winery–Marsha is here today. We will drive over an hour each way, probably spend the afternoon at Jeanne's, and get Fred into a bed at Fox Chase in the early evening, getting home by 9 or 10 p.m. It's just how it goes.

And it does go that way. Fred was upset–they were treating him like a child. The registration desk called me his daughter. After the nurse sees us in triage, we wait until she comes to take Fred to an examination room to get him ready for the doctor. Then they will come to get me. I look at Fred and say nicely, "I think I better come along." Reluctantly, she says, "Yes, but the doctor may not like this." I've heard it all. We get him to the room, and the nurse explains that Fred needs to give a urine sample and asks if we've used these cups before. They have three wipe pads you can use to clean yourself three times before peeing a little and then peeing into the cup. She's looking at Fred, and I say, "I don't think you understand. We are here to get him admitted to Fox Chase. He can barely hold a pen, let alone go through all that." Fred gathers himself up and says, "Bullshit," as forcefully as possible. He then says, "We want to see the doctor." "OK," she says. The other nurse who came in slips out. The doctor is Russian and says he needs to do some simple tests, as Fox Chase requires. Fred says he doesn't want any; they have never asked him for a urine sample, and he can't go. The doctor says, "That's OK, we'll put a catheter in." "NO," says Fred emphatically. I try to moderate, and finally, the doctor says he will call Dr. Wallace, who's on call. I say, "Yes, we have already talked to him." We continue to wait, and the doctor returns and says to talk on the phone with Dr. Wallace, who explains again in detail why they need to perform some basic analysis to determine what type of care Fred needs. I say, "Why don't you just call Dr. Cheng? He wanted Fred in the hospital ten days ago." In the end, they activate his port, draw blood, and give him a chest x-ray. The doctor examines Fred and says he has about a gallon and a half of liquid in his abdomen. He calls it something like ikstatic—either a protein problem, a liver problem, or the cancer. After the test results are in, they say his potassium level is low and give him a potassium drink. Everything else was to be expected, so probably it's the cancer causing the fluid buildup. It's pressing on his intestinal system, making eating almost impossible. "How do I eat?" Fred asks. "Maybe a J-tube. Your doctors will decide. They can draw off the liquid, but it will come back."

So we get him into a room; his roommate is coughing a lot, and his caregiver is reading to him. The resident doctor comes in to review the prescription list we had prepared and examine Fred. Dr. Diaz was very nice. She asks about his age, and Fred responds, "54 going on 85." She smiles, and he keeps up his best behavior. She confirms the water in his abdomen and wants to know which nutritional drinks he likes. I look at him as he says he hates them, then he rethinks and says he likes the fruit Boost. She talks about a shaky something and says that her patients all like it or say it's OK. I hold his hands for a while and find a TV station with pictures of birds and soft music. His roommate has lung cancer, and the wife is reading aloud to him all evening. His machines go off frequently, and the nurse and aids are going in and out. The patient is loud and nervous. The wife leaves, and as she walks away from her husband's bed, her expression changes and takes on a look of pain and grief. It feels familiar to me. After a while, I leave, taking note of his room telephone number. I stop at the nurse's station, exchange telephone numbers, and check on tomorrow's CT scan appointment.

Monday, January 26, 2004

It's slow in the morning, with 3 inches of snow on

top of the ice. I drive the car up and down the driveway to pack the snow down a little and talk to Fred—he sounds good and is finally getting some rest. I'm getting ready to go to the hospital and am swimming—I don't see Fred's fish on the wall yet in the pool. Faith comes to me as I get nervous about the test results and fight not to think about anything. It is easier to have faith.

Fred looks better; he's had the CT scan; there's no news; he has eaten some lunch and is working on a very small nutritional drink, the Mighty Shake, which has 200 calories. I brought him a pile blanket to cover him up; he wants to adjust his position and fix the pillows. We decide to send home the clean down booties. There are flowers in the vase from Jen, Sean, and Olivia. I hold his hand, he squeezes my hand periodically, and I tell him little things about my day and the animals. Tashie wanted to send one of her toys along; she put one by the bag I was packing. He smiles. I mention a few of the Golden Globe results. I take his dinner tray out in the hall and happen to see Dr. Cheng. He claims he hasn't seen the CT scan results and will go look for them. I say, "We can wait till tomorrow." He says " Then we'll talk about options." I try not to read anything between the lines. I leave at about 7 p.m.

Tuesday, January 27, 2004

The Telling Day. We're expecting an ice storm and 6 inches of snow. I will go early to the hospital. Fred just called in a panic. He says, "Do you know anything?" I say, "No. What are you asking about—the test results?" He says, "Yes." He couldn't sleep all night. I ask, "Has Dr. Cheng been in?" He replies, "No, but the residents have and were talking about how to get rid of some of the liquid." I say, "OK, that's good." I tell him about the expected snowstorm and that I will get there as fast as possible. "Safely," he says. "I love you," we both say.

The internal resident removes a liter and a half of liquid. It takes a while. First, they try a needle on the right side, then, after about a half hour, on the left side—that starts flowing right away. I comment to the resident that she had said she would access the left side and then proceeded to access the right side. I try to press on the abdominal area to force the liquid out. That's about 3 pounds or ¼ of the estimated liquid weight. He feels a little better. The resident talks about the CT scan and how taking readings with all the liquid is hard. Dr. Cheng will review it again with the radiologist who read his last CT scan. Fred's mom has called twice in the last two days, wondering if we're all right. Jen thinks she's suspicious. After listening to the social worker say to the roommate that it's important to be honest with those close to you because they have a right to know, Fred says, "Maybe it's time to tell my parents." "Yes," I say, suggesting that Jen go to their house and be present when he calls. "That's a good plan," says Fred. Before I leave, Fred gets up to urinate. He has been standing for quite some time. Finally, he sits down, then gets up and says his robe is wet. I look for another and go to the nurse's aid. When I return, I inspect him and find everything wet—his clothes, the bed, and the floor. He's embarrassed. I go back and find the nurse's aid, then try to help him change into dry clothes. The hospital staff handles this like normal business.

On the way home, I call Kathy. I'm upbeat, and we

laugh about the stuff of life. She talks about how good I sound—probably relief at not being responsible for Fred's care right now.

Wednesday, January 28, 2004

9 a.m.: I call his room, and we chat about how he is. He says, "OK. Dr. Cheng came in last night and said the CT scan was the same." I ask, "What about the fluid?" He says, "He didn't say." I say, "Well, I guess that's good news. We hoped for better, but that's still good news." He says, "Yes. When are you coming to the hospital?" I say, "I will leave around 1 p.m., so I should be there around 4 p.m." He says, "OK." We both say, "I love you."

4 p.m.: Traffic is slow because of the snow and ice. I call his room to say I am running late. He is extremely upset. I ask, "Why?" He says, "Guess." I ask, "Did Dr. Cheng say something?" He replies, "No, but he wants to see both of us." Alarms go off as I search my brain for other clues. I ask, "The roommate?" He replies, "Yes." I ask, "Has he been talking all the time?" He says, "Yes, it's been constant, and people are in and out constantly; I've gotten no sleep." I say, "I am hurrying. He says, "Well, Cheng has been waiting for you and said he'd see us tomorrow." I feel panic rising from my legs up. I say, "I'll call the nurses' station; we'll get you moved, and Cheng must still be there; he's in the clinic; he has to see us today." I call the nurses' station and tell them about the room: "Do you know what's been happening in the room?" I ask. They reply, "No, but we only have a female bed. And we must speak to Dr. Cheng today." I say, "OK." I call Fred as I get to Fox Chase, and he says Cheng will be there around 5:15.

When I reach the room, Fred reaches out to me in relief. He says they are moving him. I say, "Good. Do you want to sit in the hall?" He replies, "Yes," so we move outside the room to wait for Dr. Cheng. An hour later, they say he is coming. I help move his stuff to the new room. His gown is wet again, so I look for something. I have clean underwear, and he puts them on. He tells me his side was leaking–that's why everything is wet. The aid figured it out when he told her they put a needle in his right side too, which was sore. So now both sides have a bag attached to catch the fluid still draining. "For now, you have no roommate; maybe you'll get a night alone." That is not to be. Ten minutes after we get Fred in bed, his new roommate is wheeled in. Dr. Cheng finally arrives, and we sit in the hall. He says the liquid has live cancer cells, which is a disease progression, even though the CT scan showed the tumors were the same. Fred is weaker than he was ten days ago and thinks it may be the cancer, not just the chemotherapy. He talks about the options: go to rehab to try to build him up so he can take more treatment, or go home to hospice care and be as comfortable as possible. I push all emotions aside and ask whatever questions come to mind. He doesn't suspect Fred will respond to rehab, but we can try. He wants us to decide by tomorrow, and he's sorry it isn't better news. We keep ourselves composed and go back to the room. I have an overwhelming urge to leave, to run away.

Fred sits on the bed as we process this information. We don't speak. Finally, I ask, "You don't want to go to rehab?" He replies, "No." I say, "You want to go home, and there's no reason to stay at the hospital." He says he can't stay here. We can go home. Dr. Cheng says, "You can sign yourself out!" He looks at me with hope. I will go tell them.

I go to the nurse's station and find our nurse. I start to tell her that Fred wants to go home, and the tears start falling. I tell her we'll come back tomorrow to get his abdomen drained. She says she'll have to call Dr. Cheng. I wait. He calls in short order, and as she's talking to him, she gives me the phone. He says slowly that we can do that but that the hospice is set up from the in-patient perspective. I ask again, "What is hospice?" He ignores my question and continues, "Your insurance provides many services, but they must be set up as in-patient services." I say, "You have just told us that Fred will not live long—what is the timeline?" He doesn't like to say anything specifically, partly because he is always wrong and partly because a miracle could happen. He says, "A few weeks to a few months." I say, "OK, we'll stay tonight, and we want his abdomen drained tomorrow. When will he be ready to go?" He says, "They can get everything set up in one day, but it takes all day." I say, "OK, I will come late in the afternoon." He says, "Yes, that's good."

I go back to the room. Fred is expecting to leave and is upset when I tell him he has to stay. He is in deep emotional pain. I get the nurse to bring some Ativan. I ask, "Do you want me to stay?" "Yes," he says. And I think about how it's not good for me, and "how can I arrange for someone to take care of Tashie? It's almost 9 p.m." I hold his hand for an hour and get the nurse to bring two Percocet, hoping he will calm down a bit. He doesn't want me to leave, but I say, "I must, and I will call you first thing in the morning." I feel guilty as I leave.

I call Mom and Kathy on the way home. I have no feelings. I feel like I am walking in space. This can't be real. It's just not possible.

Thursday, January 29, 2004

I get through to Fred, and he asks, "When are you coming?" I say, "In a little while. What did they do in ultrasound?" He says, "They took out 14 lbs of fluid." I say, "14 lbs of fluid! How do you feel?" "Lighter," he says, and I smile.

Kathy and I leave at about 3 p.m. We get to the room,

and he is anxious but quiet. We sit and wait. The nurses come and go, and the home care and discharge nurses come to talk and give me papers to sign or instructions. I ask about the physical therapy and "how does that get started?" She ignores me and talks to Fred, saying, "All you need to do is get up and walk around each day—normal activity. The goal is to make you comfortable."

Kathy goes to get her car. Fred walks to the car from the entrance and the nurse comments on how good that is. At home, Fred is anxious to eat. I open a bottle of champagne, and we spend a quiet evening deep in our thoughts. The hospice social worker calls, and we have an introductory conversation. I ask, "Have you seen a miracle?" "Lots," she says as she tells me about her mother, which is similar to Dave's story. I believe. They will come tomorrow.

Friday, January 30, 2004

I got up twice to check on him last night. The hospice social worker calls, and I tell her we don't want them to come today. "Tomorrow?" she asks. I say,

"Yes, OK." I try to be upbeat, but Fred is morose all day. I tell him the hospice social worker's story about her mother being diagnosed with cancer in her fifties, being told she wouldn't live, and then going into remission one year later and living another 25 years. "That's pretty good," he says.

At night, he is angry with me and wants to know why I didn't stay in the hospital with him on Wednesday. He says, "You said you would, and then you left." He talks for ten minutes about how bad it was. I say, "I'm very sorry, but I had to come home; it was late, Tashie couldn't be left alone, and I didn't know if I could get someone to stay with her." He looks at Tashie. It's gut-wrenching and heartbreaking. The truth is, I didn't want to stay; I wanted to run away. Later, I tell him I will not leave him; he's not alone; he is here, at home.

Jen calls, and we talk about her going down to Cape Cod to tell his parents. She plans on going on Saturday. Fred nods and is thankful that Jen will do the telling.

Saturday, January 31, 2004

I can't move or think. It feels like I am being pulled through a meat grinder. I don't think I can survive the day. I call Kathy and break down on the phone while leaving a message. Can she please come down? I don't think I can talk with the hospice people alone. Then I think, "Oh no, one of her children may get the message." I feel bad that they may be upset. I finally get moving. I go to the pool and also buy groceries. Unbelievably, Fred wanted sushi yesterday and coleslaw. I get back just before noon. The nurse pulls in after me. Confusion! I am in the winery and think she's a customer, so I wait in the winery. Then I finally realize it and run to the house—she's already there, and Fred looks at me like, "You left me alone again!"

The nurse gets started, and then the social worker arrives. It's a bit of a tag-team approach, with everyone feeling their way. They go through the mounds of papers; we discuss available services, and I like the sound of the aids twice a week for two hours. They check Fred's vitals, and we go over the prescriptions. Some are covered by Hospice 100%. That's one of the selling features—100% medical coverage. It's really a managed-care approach. I talk Fred into getting a bedside commode for when I'm not around; we can keep it downstairs. "Is this OK with you, Fred?" I ask. He says, "This is all new, and we'll just have to see how it goes." The visitors nod and repeat that nothing is irreversible. They talk about emergency supplies and stay a long time doing their paperwork. I think they should go away sooner; they can do their paperwork somewhere else. It's been almost three hours, and we haven't eaten lunch. I'm tired, and my mind is mush. Before they leave, the social worker asks the "tough question": Have you talked about your funeral arrangements? I look at Fred and say no, and that we have never talked about it—I don't know what he wants. Fred says nothing. Finally, they leave and pat my shoulder before going out the door.

I can barely think, and we still have Fred's parents to talk to. We get food and sit quietly to eat. My body grinds to a halt. I sit with a blank stare. There is not enough energy to think about talking with Mary and Tisch. Thankfully, dusk descends.

Sunday, February 1, 2004

I tell Fred I can't stand that we are not sleeping in the same room. He asks, "What am I supposed to think about?" I say, "What? When?" He replies, "My last moments." I am not ready for this. "I don't know," I say. He says, "What do people do? There is no future for me. Why should I care about anything?" I say, "But maybe we're jumping the gun." He says, "That's what hospice is—the button." I say, "The button?" He says, "Yes, the pain button, the way out." I am speechless; agony takes over my being. I think, "Why can't he enjoy today and hope for tomorrow?" I ask, "Are you in pain?" He replies, "No, not physical pain." I say, "I hope that you can find some peace." He says, "Peace is pushing the button." He is crying now and talking about our life's work here—the vineyard and winery. He says, "We're just on the verge of something significant, and I won't be here." Recognition of the 13 grueling years we spent outside daily tending the vines or doing cellar work, working as slave laborers, having a vision for the industry, pushing change, and working the land to hope for a livelihood one day. Yes, this is a bitter pill to swallow. He kicked around in various jobs for years; his previous marriage failed. At 40, we landed here and put our entire beings into making it work. We both sweated equity; his soul will walk the vineyard. It cannot be found anywhere else. I say, "We have recognition: the Paris medals! No other winery in the East has them, and none in the US or anywhere outside of France has a Paris Gold for champagne. You are in the history books." It is not enough; he wants to live.

Monday, February 2, 2004

I get up early and wake Fred up by accident. He didn't sleep well and wants to move downstairs. He only got up once during the night, and he has trouble getting up from the bed, so I have to help pull him up. We settle him into the La-Z-Boy, and I go to the kitchen. I must write this all down; the last few days have been confusing, and this helps me sort it out. But I don't have time to write, as Fred wants me to be with him. I can't go forward unless I write about the last four days.

I tell Fred I don't feel this is right; I don't believe

this is the end. I rush to the pool and run errands. In the pool, I feel strongly that maybe we're reading too much into hospice. He can recover and get more treatment. I'll work to make him strong again. We must go on and never give up; it's not over till the fat lady sings the blues. I feel better. Hope is much easier. I have realized this before. That is probably why so many are successful at selling hope. It's easier for the patient, the caregiver, and the medical staff.

I have lunch, then go to a PPWG meeting at another vineyard. We must talk about the strategy for the Quality Program. I frequently communicate my schedule to Fred and call him several times from the road. We re-establish our telephone code: one ring, then call back. He is in better spirits today. Mary, Fred's mom, calls around dinner time. His mom is named Mary, and mine is Mary Ann, and their birthdays are days apart in September. She has questions like, "Do you think the vineyard chemicals were the culprit?" I say, "No, they have told me that the thinking is genetic predisposition." I tell her about the beginning when he was in the emergency room, and the doctor asked if there was cancer in the family. She says, "And he didn't know." I say, "Right, he didn't know." She says, "Well, there are lots, "My father died of pancreatic cancer, my mother of throat cancer, my grandfather of pancreatic, my brother of brain cancer, and my uncle of throat cancer." I am speechless.

Tuesday, February 3, 2004

Martha, the nurse, is coming around noon today. I will teach Miguel today how to do my job of champagne disgorgement this morning; hopefully, he and Dave will work on that. God bless Dave. I am still mad at Fox Chase; how can they not have something to help Fred? Fred is worried about the vineyard spraying and is talking with me about that. We get out all the literature, and I order the current spray schedule from Cornell. I am still trying to find time to finish the solar grant application. Another day goes by. I leave at 2 p.m. to run errands, go to the pool (always the pool), and to the pharmacy contracted for hospice prescriptions–a 40-minute one-way trip–managed care–good for them but not for the caregiver. I return Pastor Cindy's call while driving and give her our bad news. We talk about dealing with this bad news, whether we accept it or not. She talks about her belief in another life in heaven. It is much easier if you believe in another life.

Tears flow freely again.

"Can't you make him well?" I say, looking skyward.

When I get home, I show Fred all the food items and pretend we are planning a nice evening together. Fred eats well but is then uncomfortably full. He may have to vomit, but he sits for a while. After I go to bed, he comes upstairs to the bathroom. I didn't know he was constipated—the downside of pain medications. He's so upset later that he won't take the Percocet and has a bad night.

Wednesday, February 4, 2004

Hope is for the caregivers to keep us going.

I sit with Fred all day as he discusses spraying issues, equipment, philosophies, chemicals, schedules, the quirks of our vineyard, and how to handle the slope. He's worried that I won't be able to do it. The Home Medical Supplies truck arrives at noon—nice young men going in and out carrying the bed upstairs, an oxygen unit, tanks, and a walker. They are about to bring in a 100-pound tank of oxygen when I say, "Wait a minute—do we need that? He's not on oxygen; this is just a precaution." They say, "Well, you'll have to pay $45 to have it delivered if you don't take it now." I question the other items, and finally, he agrees that we should just keep the 4-hour portable tank. They try to put everything in the living room, and I have to work to get it spread out and not in the living room. We're trying to live without constant visual reminders. Finally, they leave, and I get Fred lunch. We talk again about spraying, and then I leave for the pool and groceries. Dinner is quiet; Jennifer is coming tomorrow. I still have not started cleaning. I sit down with a pair of scissors and remove the Zofran RX from its plastic casing. Two pills are packaged as samples. One hundred pills—it takes me 30 minutes to open up all the sample packages and put them in a bottle. Hospice may be compassionate care, but it is also about managing costs.

Thursday, February 5, 2004

I go out in the morning, after Fred, and I go over some vineyard stuff. Home at noon, get Fred lunch, check the winery, and the nurse is here already. She measures his girth at 45 inches. She has called Anne about scheduling a drain. What hospital do we want to try? She calls Anne, and they discuss how to set this up. I ask, "Will it make a difference where we go?" She says, "No." We talk about the bed with a nice air mattress, but it needs a motor to run constantly, and it vibrates the floor. Fred only slept in it for a couple of hours. Did she know it required a motor? She is very gentle and peaceful in her style. We don't hurry our conversations. Fred decides to give it another try. Martha had called this morning and given me a list of anti-constipation stuff to get, and she asks about that. Then we go over the emergency kit, and she writes down directions. Once in a while, I wonder if they really think we will need all this stuff: oxygen, morphine suppositories, and other fast-acting pain medications. Of course, he always says he is not in pain. But last night, he was "uncomfortable," and I gave him a Percocet in the early evening. Jen arrives and listens to some of the conversation. She goes to the kitchen. I tell her she can come in and meet the nurse. She joins us, and it feels normal that she is with us. Fred's been groggy all day from the extra Ativan. When I take Fred up to the bed, his legs are so thin and light as I help tuck him into the hospital bed. But it's so nice that we are sleeping in the same room. I can easily check on him. This is the first day I acknowledge that we are in the hospice phase—a phase you never want to be in.

Hospice

Friday, February 6, 2004

It's so nice to have Jen here; it feels like we are whole. We have to go to a local hospital for the first time since the diagnosis, for an abdominal drain. The roads are wet, and flooding is happening everywhere since the ground is frozen. We get to the hospital in time; Jen gets Fred in a wheelchair, and I park the car. But they can't find the appointment. We get the usual runaround for twenty minutes, sending us one place after another. I calmly tell the receptionist, "Please look again; we have an appointment." I repeat this several times, and finally, after a few calls, they locate the appointment. Jen says, "You're very good at this; I would be losing it." I say, "The first thing you learn is patience." The waiting area is not very wheelchair friendly, so we wait in the hall. Fred nods off. I go to find someone concerned with the crowd in the waiting room. They look at me and try to dismiss me quickly with a "we're all very busy." I stand there and say, "I have a patient waiting in the hall." They ask, "Who is it?" I reply, "Fred Maki." A kind nurse stops, comes to me, and says, "Where is he?" We walk back to where he and Jen are waiting. The nurse looks at Fred, who is slumped over in the chair, and nods. "We'll be with you shortly." Tears are welling up, and I move away, so Jen doesn't see me crying. I walk the halls for a few minutes to get my composure back. "Keep your head up high" plays in my brain.

They arrive shortly and take Fred. The nurse assumes he will go alone, and I say twice that I will come with him. He wants me to stay during the procedure. The nurse isn't sure what the doctor will say, but he says fine. They take off 6 liters, and it comes off in about 45 minutes. It's pink; I guess he is bleeding inside. I don't really know, and I don't want to ask. The doctor talks about not wanting to take off more than 8 liters, as it is a shock to the system. That's probably why he was so exhausted last weekend. We get home easily, and Fred enjoys the ride—lots of water and flooding. He has a pretty good night's sleep and sleeps until 8 a.m. I get Jen up because she is leaving today. During breakfast, she goes to the kitchen. I find her crying, and we hug and cry together a little. She talks about how sad and unfair it is. Later, we sit with Fred, and she gives him a beaming smile. He loves her very much. It is good for both of them to be together, and for me too. She leaves for her flight at 11:30, and I go out; same drill. In the afternoon, Fred says how nice it was to have her visit. She will come again soon. In the afternoon, the nurse comes again to check on him after the procedure. She measures him at 38 inches; he was 45 inches before the procedure. He looks better. I allow myself to think that somehow he is better.

Monday, February 9, 2004

Kathy comes to visit on her way to Westtown Friends School to visit her children, Katy and Tyler. I tell Fred she will only be here for a short while. We stay in the kitchen and have tea. I tell her everyone's been calling and wants to come to visit. I realize many people feel compelled to call and visit because of their needs. And all the hospice people are calling and want to come help. Fred doesn't want anyone to visit. We've always been independent and self-sufficient. We have the nurse three times a week, the hospital once a week for the drain, and I have a lot to do here, the bare minimum, to keep things going. She understands and suggests telling them they can come to clean the windows. (Good idea!) It's always been a struggle to maintain space for Fred, and now it feels like we're running out of time. I don't want anyone here, either.

Tuesday, February 10, 2004

Everyone is calling. The pressure to come here is overwhelming. Cindy wants to come out. Dad calls and says he is taking a ride out. I need time, precious time, to call everyone back. Anne calls right as I am leaving. I tell her I'm not mad at them anymore. She asks, "Mad or angry?" I reply, "I'm angry and disappointed that they can't help Fred anymore." She talks about how it doesn't make sense to do any more chemotherapy—he'd have to be in bed. It's about quality of life. Now maybe he can have some quality. I can tell he can eat well and feels better now that the fluid has been removed. She says maybe he can sustain himself enough that he may stay at this place for a while. I say, "He hopes he's around to see the new shoots come up." She says, "He should make that; it's March, right?" "No, it's late April or early May." Ummmm, and silence is all I get. I tell her to say hi to Dr. Cheng and tell him Fred's doing great, and we're still waiting for the cure. As we hang up, there is no response. I have to go to the hospice pharmacy again, 40 minutes each way. Martha, the nurse, will be here around 2:30 to 3 p.m. Dad insists that he will feel better if he comes for a visit. The needs of the living somehow balance the needs of the dying. I'm losing the struggle. I agree that Dad can come and tell Fred I'm sorry. He says, "OK." I check on the team in the winery and rush off to get back in time. I check on Fred by phone; he sounds OK. I get home at 2:35 p.m. Dad pulls in ten minutes later. I go to the kitchen to get tea, and Fred asks Dad to sit awhile, then Martha pulls in. We're all in the living room, and Dad says he'll go to the kitchen; Fred says it's OK. Martha checks his vitals; he measures 42 inches. I believe the fluid is accumulating slower, but not by much. We discuss constipation, new prescriptions, and using the walker. I get it out, and she has Fred do a few tries at getting up out of the chair. She reviews the medications and asks, "Is he sleeping?" I comment that we probably should have had a hospital bed for the last year—he's had to sleep in the La-Z-Boy. His ankle and foot swelling have decreased since he started using the bed. She comments on how it looks better. Martha is surprised that Fred only takes a few Percocet pills every day. His bowels start growling, and he gets up quickly to go upstairs. No, we don't have a downstairs bathroom, but there is a commode. We discuss using a privacy screen to make an area downstairs for the portable commode. Before he comes back, she says she is anticipating that he will need more pain medicine and wants to ensure we have enough. It's one of those looks and messages that stop me cold. She's preparing me for the next step. I don't want to go there. Finally, she leaves, and Fred acts like he wants to be alone. I walk Dad to his car. When I return, Fred is upset that Dad sat through his exam; it should be private! I say, "But you said he could stay." He says, "I know, I was trying to be polite." I say, "I'm so sorry; everyone wants to come, and I'm trying to keep your peace. I'll try harder." He wants me to sit with him. The phone rings incessantly. Finally, I pick it up; it's the volunteer coordinator. She asks if this is a good time. I tell her I am overwhelmed; I had asked that she call, but now it is just too much. Everyone is calling and wants to come visit. We are private people, and I'm struggling with it all. She says we are special people, and everyone's love is pouring out on us. They want to give us love. This helps me, and I tell Fred something like that. Everyone means well – they just want us to feel their love.

Later, Fred says that he can stand up better today.

Wednesday, February 11, 2004

I can hardly move. Everything seems enormously difficult. I have to return to the hospice pharmacy and pick up his medications. I am giving him his medications – a group in the morning with Milk of Magnesia to help with regularity, and then a group at night. I also give him extra Ativan and Percocet in the middle of the night. We are having much better nights, and at least I know what he is taking and when. This relieves him also, so I imagine.

Today I went to the drive-in window so I wouldn't be embarrassed. It was OK. The swelling in his feet and ankles is definitely going down. The hospital bed is making a big difference. We should have had one since his surgery. He has had to sleep in the La-Z-Boy because he can't lie down. Fred is not feeling well tonight; he gets sick eating dinner. He throws up in little batches. He won't take the anti-nausea suppository. I discover what one of the pills is—the same as one of the emergency suppositories. I give him Zofran, the new drug, and Lorazepam (Ativan). He calms down. These episodes worry me. I assume the cancer has just taken another chunk of his life. Later, he has two cookies and some juice before bed. He needs more Percocet tonight.

Thursday, February 12, 2004

The hospital called late yesterday; they have to reschedule Fred's appointment. I am concerned that this will be their way, and I question the weekly schedule. We have to leave quickly for our 10:30 a.m. appointment. I have to call and cancel other things for today. On the way to the hospital, Fred asks, "Why do I have to have a commode? Why do I have to have the suppositories? Why do I have to have the walker? Why do I need a wheelchair? And why do we need the oxygen?" I answer each question with, "It is only for convenience," and discuss different situations. "It's an insurance policy; you probably won't need them." He listens closely to my answers.

Fred tries to walk into the hospital but gets stuck going around the car. I rush to get a wheelchair, which is thankfully just inside the entrance, and get him in it. I have left the car running at the entrance, so I push him inside and run out to move the car. We should use the valet next time.

When I check in at the hospital, they ask the same questions as last week. I tell them it's the same; don't they have the info from last week? The receptionist is the same person. He says he will save some of the information, then asks for a diagnosis. I look him in the eyes and say, "Cancer," and he replies, "What kind?" They make me relive it again, "Esophageal!" Then he stops asking, gives me the printout, and sends me to the next receptionist.

They only draw off a little over three liters. When it starts running, I am alarmed by the much darker red color than last week. The doctor is also concerned and continues to ask questions. We give little in response, not wanting to open our wounds. She will send it for analysis for bacteria—a possible infection. Finally, I give her Anne's name and number. I am afraid we will constantly be asked questions. Fred and I talk in the car on the way home about not wanting to tell them the whole story.

At night, I leave Anne a message about giving out her name and number and the alarmingly blood-colored liquid. Can they do anything to stop the internal bleeding? I am propelled to act on the passing thought that maybe I am missing something.

Don't give up... Never give up. "Don't give up," I can still hear my parents say.

Friday, February 13, 2004

Today Dave and Dave Jr. are coming, and we will

have an outside day. We'll clean up tree debris from all the wind storms this year, and this is preparation for the tree line clean up at the top property line. We've been here for 13 years, and things have been growing into the vineyard space. The gypsy moths and other critters are becoming bigger pests. Fred would have done this himself over time, but he has not been well for several years. We discover the chain saw doesn't really work and decide on a new one. We make the purchase over the phone, and Dave will pick it up on his way. Dave is comfortable with chain saws; he has a wealth of experience from the military service and his manufacturing background. We are blessed that he is working with us and wish we could pay him more.

When I return from my outing, they are ready to ignite this huge pile. They have worked hard and, in less than two hours, have a pile to make a pyre. I order lunch, and then the nurse arrives. Martha's boss is here today with someone in training. I run in and out to check on the team and talk with Diane. It sounds mostly like a review. I dash out several times, getting a walnut branch cut down, something I've wanted to do for years. It's holding the weeping cherry down. The tractor gets stuck going uphill. The ground is soft, wet, and has a slushy, frozen cover. The big wheels start spinning. I'll try it, but we have to take the cart off. I dash back in to check on the visitors and give Fred a walkie-talkie. The sun is shining, and I want to be outside; I'm sure Fred does too. After the nurses leave, I realize the flowers, gift card, and jewelry box must be for me! Dave must have brought them. They're not signed, and I look at Fred and realize he was supposed to sign them. I give him a pen, and he makes it official. "Happy Valentine's Day!" I give him kisses and hugs. Later, I thank Dave and Jenny. How sweet of them! It turns out that on Tuesday, when I wasn't around, Dave talked to Fred about getting them for him. What a nice surprise! The delicate bracelet has a lovely heart, and I wear it in the evening. When Dave leaves, we put up the barricade, and then I have to lie down because I'm so tired. At night, we watch Lord of the Rings. The adventure begins. We have this weird thing going on between the DVD player, DirectTV, and our TV. Switching back and forth almost always causes the TV system to 'hang up' in computer terms.. After taking a break, I spend

30 minutes trying to get it back on. Oh well.

Saturday, Valentine's Day, 2004

"Never give up; keep on going," I say to myself as I get up each day. It's my new motto. He's alive and eating. I will try to keep it that way.

Sunday, February 15, 2004

Mom comes to visit. Fred is morose. We make truffles. I decided yesterday to make them for the winery. I'm disappointed in most chocolates, so I will experiment. Then we take Tashie for a walk in the woods. We can only do that in the winter when the fields are not being worked. It's her winter treat and keeps her from being house-happy. She is careful to stay only so far ahead and pick the path for us. I am blessed every day that she is in my life.

After lunch, I take Mom to the Y, where she sits in the whirlpool and walks in the pool while I swim. She is a little slower and has fallen twice this winter. I need to look for those cleat pull-ons for her.

Fred ate a little lunch but has been quiet and moody.

He says he's happy I'm home. He doesn't want to eat. I try to baby him a little. He prefers when visitors do not take up my attention. We watch *Two Towers*, and he goes to the bathroom and doesn't come down. I go up to check, and he is constipated again and struggling. For the next hour, he struggles. Up and down, he can't go. Finally, he does a little, but now that he is worn out and short of breath, he returns to the bed, can't speak, and hangs his head down. He stays like this for a long while. Finally, he takes a drink. I put the pills in his mouth, one by one, and then he slides into bed, hot and uncomfortable. He eventually falls asleep and wakes up refreshed.

Monday, February 16, 2004

He groans that Jeannine, the PT, is coming at 8:30 a.m. He rallies and takes a shower; I lay out clean clothes. He talks with her and is involved. He shows her his picture from two years ago: "That's what I looked like before." She asks about his treatments, and we are vague. She comments that it's good that he's done chemotherapy—good to get that done. He gets up and walks quickly—beyond where he really is. She checks his strength—legs, feet, arms. They conclude that his main complaint is weakness. What is his goal? Probably to see what he can do. She starts with her paperwork. I go in and out with chores. At a point, she is checking his insurance, Personal Choice, and I say, "He's on hospice," and I look at her. She says, "Yes," matter-of-factly. I wonder, are there different hospice definitions? I remember the shock of seeing his insurance benefit approval form—there it was in black and white: terminal hospice. I have hidden that form from all eyes. It feels evil when I think of it.

We will never give up.

Tuesday, February 17, 2004

I had a restless night and have been sleeping a lot—10 hours/night. I'm concerned about wine competitions: what should I enter, and is anything good enough? I have outthought myself many times before. Fred helps me keep a balance. We work as a team. I depend on his participation. What if he doesn't make it? We have done everything as a team. French Creek

Ridge Vineyards is about both of us. I go forward and assume there is hope. It may be the only way I can go forward. Confusion reigns in my brain today. I have an uneasy feeling that something is happening or that I am not doing something I should. What am I missing? This journal is becoming my running dialogue with myself.

Wednesday, February 18, 2004

I am pretending that Fred will live and that, somehow, we will go on. The evidence is growing against this.

And the patient is...

Growing weaker, thinner, and quieter.

I chatter away, cheery, talking about the day's news.

Slightly more shortness of breath.

Sallow and pale,

But eating.

"Is he eating?" Everyone asks.

Thursday, February 19, 2004

Today we will have a hospice volunteer while I am out for about four hours. The volunteer is our neighbor, which is a surprise to us. Fred doesn't want anyone, of course. Finally, I say, "It's for me, so I don't have to worry about you while I'm out of the house." "OK," he says with a nod. I show the volunteer around and tell her what Fred should have for lunch. She is gracious and expresses how sorry she is to Fred. He only wants to be alone. I wonder how things will go. I leave my cell number on the table with his medications. After I leave, I think of all the things I should have told her about. I reach for my cell phone and find I have left it at home. It's too far to go back now. I deliver wine for the new Starwine competition, pick up a non-holiday ribbon, and stop at a pay phone to call Fred. He doesn't respond; no one does, and there is a brief moment of terror that something has occurred. Finally, Fred picks up; he was in the bathroom. It was a big effort to go upstairs and downstairs. He's OK, and I say, "I'll be home soon." I grab a few groceries, and I feel distracted all day. We eat in silence. My back has been sore all week; I take a little extra muscle relaxer and fall asleep on the floor at 9 p.m.

Friday, February 20, 2004

Fred is uncomfortable and has been up four times during the night. I get up at the slightest stir. The fear of his last breath is always with me. At 6:30 a.m., he is awake in the La-Z-Boy. We have an early breakfast, and I dash to the pool, for there will be no time later. At 10:15 a.m., I get Fred into the car and head to the county hospital. This time we use the complimentary valet parking. They have wheelchairs right by the entrance. Fred doesn't object today; a wheelchair is what he assumed. The receptionist gives me the runaround – "Where's your paper?" I say, "We don't have any." She says, "I can't do anything without your paper." I say, "We have an appointment; you can check his name." She says, "I can't do anything without the paper – and where's your RX?" I say, "They have it in the department; we come every week." She says, "Well, you'll just have to go to the department and get the paper. I need the paper; I can't do anything without it." She asks, "What department?" I say,

"Radiology: an ultrasound test." She says, "Are you sure it isn't the Oncology department?" That's the limit of my patience. I look around and find the male receptionist that has checked us in the last two times and approach him—in the next cubicle. He acknowledges me and starts working on the computer. I give him Fred's name, the doctor's name, and the diagnosis again. I step away to bring Fred around to this side. When I return to the check-in counter, the first person I encountered is blabbing in a loud voice to the male receptionist, "Well, she didn't have any papers, and I need the papers, so I told her to..." I finally can't take it and say to the wall, "I can hear everything you're saying, in case you want to know." She replies back, "That's OK," and walks away. Then we proceed to the next check-in desk and wait until they are finished chatting before handing the paper over. They ask the same questions and finally give me directions. I cut off the person and say, "I know, we're here every week." As I wheel Fred away, the other woman says, "Well!" Loud enough for me to hear.

We were never treated so poorly at Fox Chase.

Finally, we're at the last check-in point: the ultrasound department. Then we're told they're running late, and the doctor has to do a biopsy for a patient coming down from a hospital floor. I don't let the nurse escape and question how long we will wait. Then I gather enough reserves to push back. I say "Why are you doing the in-patient? They can wait. You should have called us before we traveled here if you were late," and on and on. And I ask for the person's name to give feedback to—the supervisor looks at me and says I can give that to her. I say, "No, it's not just about here; it's the whole process." In short order, the ultrasound technician comes out and says, "We're taking you into another room to get started right away." I am grumpy and on the verge of tears. I keep the scowl on my face lest I break apart. Four liters are removed, at least as much as last week, and we will keep the weekly schedule. As I wheel Fred out, he thanks everyone and extends his hand when we get close to the doctor, who moves quickly to reciprocate and touch his hand, saying, "Take care." My eyes well up with tears; I struggle to hold my head high; Fred isn't looking, and I'm still his strong but rude Janet. On the way home, he wants some deli bologna; I wait in another line while he sits in the car. I get him lunch at home, warm up some leftovers, and dash to my semi-annual back check-in appointment with Dr. Donaldson. Deedee greets me, and when she asks about Fred, I break down, and the dikes come crashing down. She wants to know what happened; Fred was doing so well. I am left alone for a few thankful moments to compose myself. Dr. D nods that he knows; he's gotten some reports. I tell him the sequence since we last talked. He offers no hope but listens. I say, "Have you ever seen a miracle?" He says "Yes, definitely." And there is absolutely no other explanation. I say, "We need divine intervention." He nods and asks if I need anything to help with sleep or anything. "I'm good," I say, wondering if something can take my pain away.

I rush home for the nurse's visit; Martha is just arriving when I get home. We have much to talk about. Fred's uncomfortable, he's not sleeping, and I'm all confused about the laxative stuff. She recommends another pain medication every 12 hours to give a better coverage base. Fred agrees. She has to call the doctor for approval. We already have some—Oxycontin pills. Fred wants to know why he is so weak. Is it the cancer? I look at Martha. She says that is a symptom of the disease's progression. We talk about his hemoglobin level. I ask, "Can he get a transfusion? Can you check his blood level?" She says, "Yes, but I need to talk to my boss." Hospice is managed care. It will pay for many things, but not treatment. I sit up and explain that we still hope things will improve; we know that no one is giving us hope, but we still have hope. She nods and says that we need to talk forthrightly about the situation. She leaves the room to use the kitchen phone, and I hold Fred's hand. He looks at me with very wide eyes–forlorn, sorry, disappointed. Will this day never end? I am so tired that I have to lie down on the couch. Martha comes back, and we try to wrap up. With cold water thrown on us, I guess pretending isn't going to cut it anymore. There's a message from the volunteer–Fred wouldn't let her give him lunch. She hopes he was all right. That figures, and he never said a word. I can't do anything now. I have to lie down for a while.

An hour later, I go to fix lox, bagels, and cream cheese and realize I forgot to buy the lox. The DirectTV is still hanging up the DVD player, and now it hangs up the TV—nothing works. Fred is calling for his dinner and to get something on the TV. I run in circles; what to do first? I order takeout sandwiches and call the TV support line. After an hour, two calls, crawling behind the TV about ten times, disconnecting everything, and then reconnecting the new connections, everything is fixed. I dash out for the subs. I feed the animals and finally sit down at 7:30 to eat and watch a movie. Fred says I did a good job. I say, "Thanks."

Today, we were:

Given the runaround,

embarassed,

humiliated,

angered,

chatted to,

looked down at;

all before they threw cold water on us.

Saturday, February 21, 2004

There's a morning rush to get out of the house and back by lunch. We watch the video again since we both fell asleep. I have cried all night and all morning when out of the house. Pretending won't help now. The end is coming.

The new neighbor comes to the winery. We have left messages about growing grapes in their field across the street. They are nice and effusive about how much they love the vineyard; it is so beautiful, and that is why they bought the house. She is a consultant who works on cancer trials. Normally, interesting things to talk about take great effort to pay attention to. I listen politely to their story. My story is hitting a big wall. My overriding sensation is that time is running out. I am painfully aware of others' needs, and they are often unaware of mine. I need to guard my time left with Fred.

Sunday, February 22, 2004

I do not feel part of this earth. How dare they tell me that he has no chance? It is true that we need divine intervention. God, you can do this. Fred deserves to live; you have certainly made him suffer enough. Or is it me that you have meant to suffer?

I take Tashie for a long walk. I try to do that on Sundays as a special treat. She is such a wonderful friend. She works the route in front and picks a safe route for me. We look out for each other. When I return, I open the door to tell Fred that I'm back and will open the winery. We make eye contact immediately, and I start talking. I practice a calm, slow, soothing speech style as much as possible. He says, "I fell over." I say, "What?" He doesn't repeat to save strength. I go inside and take off my coat and boots. I ask, "Are you hurt? Where did you fall?" He says, "In the kitchen." I ask, "What were you doing there?" No answer. Then, he says, "I got up after you left. I was coming back, and I just fell backwards, completely flat." I say, "Oh my God! You could have hit your head!" "I'm OK," he says. I say, "That must have frightened you." His eyes widen, and he says, "Yes." I sit with him, and we talk about using the walker more. He is quiet the rest of the day. I am worried when I go out.

Monday, February 23, 2004

Jeanine, the PT, is coming early—at 8:30, her phone message from last night said, which I listened to this morning. Fred is upset when I tell him and give him his 12-by-12 pill. He gets dressed and goes downstairs to get some coffee and prepare for her visit. He does his exercises for her using the walker and says he feels pretty good. I tell her about the fall, and we discuss having a third point. She will get a cane for moving around the house. We talk about being uncomfortable in bed and his body position versus being comfortable in the La-Z-Boy. She suggests a neck roll, which I already have.

I have been busy with the solar project site visit for hours. We are going to get a grant, and it is significant. He will be happy. When I am done with the visitors, I get Fred a late lunch and get ready to go out. As I enter the living room, he is trying to get his rubber boots on. I ask, "What are you doing?" He says, "Going out, I'm going to stake out the new vineyard rows." When the energy is like that, I don't push back; I just go with it. I help him push his feet into the boots, wondering if I will have to cut them off later. I insist on getting him in a coat, grab mine, and run out the door in stocking feet. As he starts walking down to the equipment storage area, I get my boots on and catch up, giving him an extra arm. He is gasping for air and has to stop twice before we get there—maybe 25 yards. He is breathing very hard, and it's not slowing. We wait at least ten minutes until he can move his legs. He looks at me with scared eyes. I look straight back without fear and support his arms. I will not take this activity away from him. He slowly moves up into the Kubota seat. I help and think ahead to getting the machine moving out of the bay. I encourage resting for a moment. He starts moving backward, and I have to get him to increase the rpms, so I can lift the claw arm off the ground. It is digging a rut as he backs up. Finally, he pauses, and I lift the arm as he pivots the machine around, and he's off. I rush to grab some tools and something to use as stakes. When he arrives at the spot, I am a little behind and rush up, so he doesn't get off. He hangs his head, gasping for air, too tired to lift his head. I measure out the distance between rows and set stakes. He looks up once and motions with his hands. I interpret the motions and adjust the line. I put the tools in the bucket and tell him to drive close to the house. He slowly moves the machine away and pauses close to the house. I help him down and support him as he walks into the house. He flops into the La-Z-Boy, panting and shaking. I work quickly to remove the boots so his feet don't swell further. He cannot speak but takes a small drink. After I put the equipment away, I sit with him as he slowly calms down. He did this, but at what cost? I am worried as I leave the house, and I cry most of the time I am out. He is certainly fading. I must call Jen tonight. I put this off over the weekend. Time is moving fast.

Jen and I discuss his status and how she should plan to return again soon. They are going to Florida this weekend. I promise to call Jen and ask Martha what timeline she sees tomorrow. I already know the time is getting short.

Tuesday, February 24, 2004

I arranged for our volunteer to come as I am going to the dentist. With other errands, I will be away for four hours. Fred is sleeping later, and I have to wake him before I go. He doesn't remember the arrangements and gets upset at the "new" news. He asks again, "Why do I need anyone in the house?" I tell him again that it's for me, so I won't worry. I call after a few hours, and he has told the volunteer to go home early. I talk with her and say, "Please wait until I call and am well on my way home." She agrees emphatically.

When I get home, the volunteer has just left, and he seems OK. I sit down and ask about lunch. Then he tells me how upset he is and how he can't get any rest. The whole time, he was shaking with nervousness. I ask about an Ativan; he just took one. The volunteer is a neighbor we don't know but occasionally communicate with. I get lunch, and the social worker calls. He starts complaining while I am on the phone. I agree that she can drop by. Then I commit to Fred that I will have her come to the kitchen only; he doesn't have to see her. And remind him about Martha's visit—more groans and anxiousness. I can please no one today. I sit with Colleen, and she points out the information in the folder about signs of dying. I say they probably pointed this out at the start of hospice, but I didn't want to go down that path. She says, "You weren't ready." I talk about balancing the needs of the living with the feeling that we're running out of time. She agrees and says that's what happens. People come out of the woodwork when it's the eleventh hour. She recommends a single communication point and maybe changing the answering machine to say, "We can't come to the phone, but we listen to the messages and appreciate your call." I ask questions, and she tells me about how things usually progress. The signs of the end are when the body's systems shut down. As she leaves the driveway, Nurse Martha pulls in.

We review the medications and discuss a replacement for the Percocet that goes with OxyContin. We have a four-hour medicine and a pill bottle with one pill left. Neither Fred nor I can remember when he took these or if they were effective. My mind wanders to a meeting in the hall with Dr. Cheng before Christmas when Fred was declining, and he wrote several prescriptions, one of which was long-acting and one of which was fast-acting. She talks about "breakthrough drugs." That makes me think of a drug that will kill the cancer; she means one that breaks through the pain. He is tired but tries to be polite. She goes to the kitchen to wash her hands, and I follow. I say I spoke with Nicole, and she told me about the information in the yellow folder that I hadn't read about the signs. I ask what the timeline is that she sees. She searches my face while I am asking, nods, and then explains that they talk in terms of hours, days, weeks, and months. They don't really know, but Fred has declined, and she would guess that it will be weeks. I watch her face as she delivers the verdict. "Weeks?" I say, and she nods. I nod and walk back to the living room. When she joins us, she gets a page and returns to the kitchen to return the call. The wait feels long, and I pick up the book, "Touching the Void," that I have started to read to us. I am reading about ice climbing, another world, when she comes back briefly to say she will call Ann about new medications. I nod. She says with a nice smile, "You're reading a book?" "Yes," I say with a smile, returning to my book. The wait is long, but we are in the Peruvian Andes with the climbers attempting Siula Grande. It is one of the worlds we have shared. Finally, all is settled on the additional medications and frequency. We are instructed once again and reminded about things you could never imagine you would need to be reminded about, and the visit is over. Jen and I talk about how I never believed the clock got started on the few to many months to live. I always believed there would be something more to do. It feels like all roads are pointing to death in a short while. I go to bed somewhat accepting our fate and with overwhelming sadness and appreciation for our time together.

Sweet Cape Cod boy,

what gifts you have given me.

And what a legacy of your making you have left me.

If only I could make it so,

we would grow old together.

Hurry, Jen.

Wednesday, February 25, 2004

He is unduly tired and worn out from yesterday. Jeanine/PT is scheduled for 9:30 a.m. At 8:30 a.m., I go to the bedroom to give him his 12-hour Oxycontin. He comes downstairs, and I tell him about the visitor.

He cringes and shakes his head. "No," he says and can barely speak. I say, "OK, I'll call her." I reach her on her cell and explain again that this is too much. I ask about the cane, and she says she'll check. I say everything's too much, and I think only one day per week is appropriate for PT. We agree on Monday, and she offers Thursday if he wants a visit. I say, "OK," knowing his answer. I have to get new medications, and Pastor Cindy is coming to hug me. I tell Fred that I know that yesterday was too much, and we don't have to have anyone come in to see him. I will see them in the kitchen, and only I will take care of him. He opens his eyes and smiles at me. There are dark circles around his eyes. He is very weak and too tired to talk, but he says, "Scallops." I know what he means—we've been checking on getting fresh Nantucket scallops from the Cape fish and lobster market near his home in Hyannis. Last week it was too cold; you can't take fish when it is 32° F. or lower.

I call and order two pounds of fresh scallops and a pound of lobster meat. The scallops cost $26/lb, and the lobster meat cost $46/lb! Fred is interested in hearing these things. I try to get him food—anything appealing. Yesterday, I went to the market and bought sushi tuna, the best I've seen in a while. I make him a plate with some aged tamari for lunch.

Cindy and I have tea and show her the information from the packet and the book Colleen left, "Final Gifts." We talk about how things are, and she nods and says, "He's dying." We talk about a funeral home, and I've been wondering how Kurt's wife is doing and about a possible service. She says it could be here—rent chairs. I say maybe in the vineyard. She thinks that's a good idea and says Fred really isn't a church kinda guy. Right. She hopes he can see there is another side to dying. Everyone hopes that the person will go in that direction. It's easier to say yes, but the truth is that Fred doesn't believe there is another life.

The hospice workers are all compassionate and have a lot of experience. I think they are a learning organization, and that makes it easier to talk with them. The nurse has pushed me to accept Fred's death. I can go there. Cindy talks with me about the funeral and the service. I think about a future when I will be happy again. But I know it is most important to be in the present, to stay here with Fred, and he deserves that also. Accepting is easier than fighting.

When I go out, I leave the portable commode nearby. When I return, the commode bucket is in the front yard. Success! He used it!

At night, I try to quickly sear the tuna, cooking only the outside and leaving the inside raw. We always wish to have it prepared this way at home, but we need a grill. Anyway, it turns out not to be too bad. I make a baked potato with sour cream, which he likes. He picks at the food and eats about half. I walk upstairs behind him; getting up the stairs is a little harder tonight. He rests on the way. No new medications tonight; Percocet continues to work well.

Thursday, February 26, 2004

He gets up on his own at night, and I don't awaken till morning. We're both sleeping in a little later. He lounges in bed as best as possible; I turn the radio on and get him a magazine and the 12-hour pain medicine. When he comes downstairs, he wants dexamethasone, which helps in the morning. I can't find the bottle. He says he put it in his pocket. I look in all the pockets, thinking, "When did he get up to do that?" I ask and get no answer. Finally, I remember putting a bottle in my purse to call the hospice pharmacy when I was out to check if the prescriptions were ready. Yes, that's it. I didn't want to think about what it would take to get a new bottle. I inform him that there will be no visitors today. We are both relieved. We enjoy some time together as I continue to read our book. I catch up on the paperwork and read a little of the "Final Gifts" book.

Martha checks in and asks if the hospital has called yet to pre-register for tomorrow. I reply, "No, not yet," and I say again that their processes and/or maybe also the computer systems need work. I say, "I have a lot of business experience, Martha, and they could easily improve." Martha has not heard me speak authoritatively before, and she pauses. Then the volunteer coordinator calls to see if we are OK with the volunteer being our neighbor. Colleen certainly shared our conversation and the discussion about possibly being too close. I tell the coordinator that our volunteer is very nice and that Fred has said that many times. And repeat that we are overwhelmed with all the support. We want the volunteer to continue with us. A little later, the hospital calls to pre-register Fred and asks all the same questions. "You have all this information," I say without rudeness. "Well, we can either go through this now or you can register tomorrow when you get here; it's your choice," she replies. I endure their inefficiencies once again.

We're watching for the Nantucket scallops and lobster meat to arrive any minute–probably right after I leave. The truck comes just as I am about to leave, carrying a treasure chest box. He wants to wait till I get back to open the box.

I have to shop for the tasting event–cheeses, crackers, and fresh fruit–for 50 people. I leave the commode near Fred and the walker. He has promised not to go anywhere. We check in by phone a few times.

Raw scallops and salt right out of the container–it can't get any better. Me. I'll wait for some to be cooked.

He needs to use the restroom at night but cannot use the commode. When we get upstairs to the bedroom, he must go immediately. Right away, it turns into a difficult hour. He is so exhausted that I can barely help him back into bed. He can't talk or move. I feel a twinge in my back and rush downstairs for more muscle relaxers. I bring fresh cranberry juice up. He still can't move, resting on the side of the bed with his head hanging down. Slowly he can flop back in bed, and I grab the neck roll, which Jeanine suggested, and it does help him be more comfortable in bed. I try to give him the new 4-hour medicine, but he insists on the Percocet. OK. Finally, he falls asleep. I get up several times to check on him and give him more medications. He is sleeping quietly when I awake at 6:30 a.m.

Friday, February 27, 2004

Hospital day. I get up early to get things ready. I go up to give Fred the 12-hour and dexamethasone pills at 7:40 a.m. He can get the rest later. He's not ready yet for breakfast. He agrees to stay in bed while I go out; I put the radio on Philly sports talk. I tell him that we'll have time when I get back for him to shower. It's been a while.

I return at 9:45 a.m. and get the shower going, thinking some nice hot water will feel good. He pauses in front of the mirror for a quick glance; he looks like a Biafran giant, pregnant with abdominal fluid. I don't get much reaction to the warm water as he takes the soap and closes the door to my offer to help—he will do the washing. He lets me dry him off as he rests from the exertion. I get fresh clothes on, and he flops on the bed. I tell him to rest until it's time to go. I've backed the car as close as possible to the front walk. It's getting warmer, but I put his warm coat on him anyway. We walk slowly to the car, arm in arm. He is quiet on the ride there, nodding off. As we get closer, he asks, "What time is the appointment?" We use the valet service, and once in the wheelchair, we bypass the front desk. Much better. The radiology check-in desk doesn't have any paperwork but takes the "recurring account number" and, with initiative, calls back to the ultrasound department instead of sending us back out front. Progress. They are ready for us and get us into the room quickly. Dr. Quinn will do the procedure again but is not quite finished with another procedure. I go down the hall to the windows to call my sister Jen about tonight. I say, "I'm thinking about staying at home with Fred; are you all right?" She says, "Yes." She and Dave can cover, but I'll need to prep her for the presentation. Finally, Dr. Quinn is ready, and this time I try to engage in small talk because I know it will make them feel better. The fluid looks bloodier, and the doctor starts asking questions like, "Is he on Epogen? Are they checking his blood levels?" A transfusion would make him feel better. They take out a little over three liters. When I mention the lobsters we just got, Fred perks up, and they comment on his reaction. We chit-chat about Maine lobsters and how they don't have to be from Maine to be called Maine lobsters. They seem relieved that things went better today and that I am not so distressed. Fred thanks them, and we take off in the wheelchair. I make calls on my cell on the way home. At 3:30ish, Martha, the nurse, arrives. I have her come to the kitchen since Fred is sleeping, and I am keeping my commitment to him to meet with everyone alone in the kitchen. We go over stuff, food—where's the cane? I tell her about Cindy's visit; I know she'll want to know. I tell her the ideas for service here and that Jen will be coming down next weekend. I tell her about the bloody fluid and Dr. Quinn's comments about a blood transfusion. She says the hospice director said they would do a blood transfusion as long as Fred can get to the hospital by himself, without an ambulance, like we do every Friday. I say, "Oh, I'll have to tell Fred." But they don't know if it will do any good—maybe a few days' relief, maybe none. I tell her that Fred's wish is to see new shoots, this year's new vines, starting to grow one more time. She asks, "When is that?" I reply, "Late April." I'm throwing out anchors for everyone. I inquire about when they will perform a transfusion and whether it can be done on the same day as the drain. She will check. She leaves around 4:30 p.m: Fred is hungry for the lobster roll sandwich. I mix up a small batch and then dash to the winery to help finish the preparations. They're off at 6 p.m., and I call Jenny to ensure everyone arrives. We finish eating and watch a video; I fall asleep. It's work staying up until 10 p.m. to meet them when they return from the gallery. Finally, we can go to bed. Fred labors as he goes upstairs. He stops several times, and getting into bed is a big effort. Finally, he calms down and nods off. He gets up once an hour, feeling that he has to urinate. I get up each time to help him to and from the bathroom. Finally, it's 6 a.m., and I can get up. I'm unsure if I got any sleep, thinking about accepting that Fred's death is close. *Hurry, Jen.*

Saturday, February 28, 2004

I figure out something to make cleaning the commode easier. I line the pail with a plastic grocery bag, checking for holes. I show Fred, and he agrees: "It's a good idea." That way, he can just throw the bag outside!

I start reading the "Final Gifts" book. It concerns nurses and hospice workers and their experiences helping the terminally ill. They have named what may be the final phase "Nearing Death Awareness." Hospice began in England in 1960, when Dr. Saunders and Dame Cicely Saunders of St. Joseph's Hospital in London proposed a new way of caring for such patients—a hospice like in the Middle Ages but organized as a peaceful place "for the care of the dying on a metaphysical journey from this world to the next." The book references Dr. Kubler-Ross's stages of dying: denial, anger, bargaining, depression, and acceptance. I read quickly to see what I have missed. Hospice is for palliative care (symptoms), not treatment of the disease. That message came through.

But I keep thinking about accepting. What am I accepting, and what am I giving up? I'm giving up the fight, the small hope that yet a miracle could save his life. It ain't over yet. What if he is simply bleeding to death? Yes, the cancer is to blame, but what if the bleeding is to blame for the increasing weakness, shortness of breath, and pain? If we get a transfusion, he might perk up and continue for a while. As I start swimming, I have an uplifting feeling. I begin to form another plan. I remember that Dr. Cheng spoke of a laser technique when surgery is impossible to target the tumors. And they must have some things that can stop the internal bleeding. A way! Am I seeing a way? Are we supposed to help ourselves? This could be the way. We will take more responsibility for ourselves. Can this work? A blood transfusion, then laser the tumor sites to stop the bleeding. And maybe radiation to the lower abdomen? He didn't have it there before.

Maybe he could live another six months. I owe it to him to try. I feel hopeful again. But I won't tell him for fear of giving false hope, a concession to the fact that we are in hospice care and that this plan may be a complete fantasy. I will try it out on Mom later. When I get home, Robear wants to chat as I get stuff out of the car. It's a lovely, sunny day. I override the strong urge to say, "I need to check on Fred, and then we can talk." He persists with a few questions, and I pause to answer. I think he wants to ask about Fred but doesn't. I try to give a little time to all those who have surrounded us in some way. After ten minutes, I open the front door, make eye contact, and say, "HI, how are you?" No reply. I turn to go get more packages, and he says, "I fell," as my eye glances around the room and finally takes in the disarray. "Oh my God," I say to myself, jumping into the room. I ask, "Are you hurt?" He says, "No, I escaped again." I take a closer look at the aftermath of the living room and hospital room things that are scattered everywhere: lamps on end, broken glass, cranberry juice everywhere, trays, tables, and stools spilled over, and Fred is quietly sitting in his chair watching me take it all in. I rush to check him for cuts, etc. I ask him, "How did you land?" "Face plant," he says. I look at the path, clear rug all the way, thank God. Then it dawns on me—it's my fault. I forgot to put the walker in front of him. He was trying to balance and use the urinal. I can see him starting to sway as I think about it. I've caught him many times already, many times on the stairs. I worry that I won't be able to catch his fall. "I'm so sorry," I say lamely. "It's my fault." After seeing that he is miraculously not hurt, I start cleaning up. I get out the oxygen. After the Monday demonstration taking the Kubota for a test drive, I made a connection between his labored breathing in general, labored breathing when climbing stairs, and oxygen deprivation at altitude. If he's losing blood, he's losing available oxygen. He was that way at the beginning when the hemoglobin was 6. I explain this to Fred, who nods as I put on the oxygen. Later, he is more recovered. I read more of "Touching the Void" to us. More mountain climbing. He tells me that the scallops would be better with a breading, so I make the rest, and we share a dish. He's eating less, and I'm pushing less. But his fluids are good. At night, it is harder to get upstairs.

He pauses several times. He leans over and begins to fall backward at one point. I counter the move and push him forward. "What are you doing?" he says, not realizing his balance is precarious. Finally, he makes the bed and is exhausted and gasping. It takes a while to calm down. He gets up every hour to urinate; I get up too.

Sunday, February 29, 2004

Leap Year! We get one extra day. He wants to come downstairs early. He has a little breakfast and wants me to stay around. I read our book for an hour and then take Tashie out. After lunch, I go shopping and swimming. I make another Romertouf dish, beef Bourguignon. Jen calls to check in, and I tell her about my ideas. I say, "I'm not trying to give Fred false hope, but maybe a little more time." She agrees that I should ask and says the doctors expect this. I lose track of what I'm cooking, and the stew gets overdone. OK with me, but not with Fred. He won't eat the meat, but the broth and vegetables are great. Well, maybe not great, but he eats them. Picky until the very end! I enjoy most of a bottle of our newest Cabernet Franc; wow! We've been waiting for the 2001 reds, and here they are. The Oscars are on; we page in and out as we fall asleep. At 1 a.m., we start the trek upstairs. I get the oxygen running in hopes of it being easier than last night. It isn't by any means. He stops several times and nearly collapses three steps from the top. I've got his full weight on me, and I'm blocking out thoughts that my back can't handle. Somehow I wrestle him up to the landing. He collapses in a heap, breathing hard in short gasps, his head hanging on his chest. He's so exhausted that he can't keep his head up. The oxygen only reaches the bedroom door. "Help me," he says. I try to pick up his upper body and half drag him to the bed. He collapses on the end of the bed, head on the mattress. He pushes himself up so his upper body is on the mattress and his legs hang out. I can't pull him anywhere. I lower the bed's top, thinking he can slide in. Somehow, we both push and tug and get him sort of in the bed. He's gasping very hard, can't talk, and has no strength for hand signals. I rack my brain for something to do. The oxygen machine is too heavy for me to move. I lie down on the bed and wait—I'm exhausted. After an hour, he is calm. I give him more medicine and juice before kissing him goodnight. We get up four more times to use the commode. He doesn't use the urinal after falling yesterday. The commode is a bigger target.

"Hurry, Jen," I say whenever I go back to sleep.

Monday, March 1, 2004

My watch says 6:40 a.m. I look for signs of breathing, yes, and he seems to be in a deep sleep, with his head slightly up and mouth wide open. I tiptoe out of the room. Tashie waits at the top of the stairs to ensure I am going downstairs—a little computer time to add to this log. So much is happening, and fast. I can hardly get it all down, and some days there is no time. Writing in this journal now feels like I am telling a story—is it Fred's or mine? And that we are in a race to the finish.

How is Fred doing? He gets up each day to face a grim existence. Each day is a struggle within the big struggle for his life. He is not giving up, and I must not either.

Martha calls, and I update her on the weekend. I start crying. I say, "I think we have to move the bed downstairs." She says, "OK, I'll call them." I remind her about the blood transfusion question for her team meeting tomorrow. She will come here around 3 p.m. tomorrow.

PT Jeanine comes, and Fred is too tired to talk. She demonstrates how to use the cane to get up and down the stairs. I think he may never go up and down again. I tell her about last night. She seems to be really surprised that he is struggling so hard. I guess he's going downhill fast. I just don't know. I rush out for shopping and swimming, then get Fred some lunch; he picks at it and needs some nausea medications. I start cleaning the living room and moving things out. I'm just finishing up at 3ish when they arrive to move the bed. Fred moves to our bed to wait. He gets to his side for the view. After they're gone, I check on Fred, who has been very relaxed and comfortable all day. He talks about the game and wants to go downstairs to watch it. Maybe I can get another TV. Problems: We just got a satellite and have only one hookup. I go downstairs to check on things and call Dr. Cheng. I leave a message that Fred has a question. I'm cleaning off our website spam when he calls around 5:40 p.m. I discuss the bloody fluid: "The doctor was alarmed last week, and the hospice director said yes to the transfusion but has no experience to tell if it will help." I ask, "What is his experience?" He replies, "It depends on the hemoglobin level." He asks, "What is it?" I reply, "No one has checked it since the last time we went to the hospital; then it was between 10 and 11." He says they recommend a transfusion if it's eight or below, and the patient will definitely feel much better. I talk about the blood in the fluid and how it seems that, "Well, is it possible that Fred is bleeding to death?" After pausing, he says, "We need to know the level first." I say, "And what about radiation to the lower abdomen?" He replies, "He says he already had radiation." I say, "Yes, but not to the lower abdomen." He says, "It's not clear where the problem is." I say, "But you said on the January CT scan that the new tumors were in the abdomen." He says, "Yes, but it's not clear what's really going on—it could be in the original area." All I can say is, "Oh, aren't there things you could do to stop the bleeding? We know that there is no hope for a cure, but to stop the bleeding would give him a better quality of life and maybe some more time." He says, "Yes, well, we can talk about that, but first we need to check his blood levels." I say, "OK, thanks."

I go to tell Fred that I have talked to Dr. Cheng and repeat the conversation about only the blood levels and possible transfusions. He says, "Thank you for asking for me," and squeezes my hand. It's such a little thing for me to do—if only I could do more.

I bring dinner up; he's so comfy he wants to stay in bed. What a surprise! He hasn't slept in our bed for about a year. He decides to stay the night—what a nice surprise! He, Tashie, and I sleep in our bed, just like old times. And that solves the problem of where I will sleep until the Twin Airbed arrives on Thursday from LL Bean. I call and leave Martha from hospice a message about my conversation and to come tomorrow prepared to draw blood.

Sleep tight, Fred! I am so thoroughly exhausted that I can't sit or lie down. Finally, I try the La-Z-Boy and fall asleep. At eleven, I go upstairs. Tashie and Fred are sleeping peacefully. It's so nice to be in our bedroom; the commode is placed on the side of the bed, so Fred just has to rotate off the bed. We get up several times at night to navigate this move.

Tuesday, March 2, 2004

He is very relaxed and stays in our bedroom all day. I check on him frequently, and he is comfortable and resting. He eats little meals, enough to keep a bird going. He has been able to sit up, pivot onto the commode at the end of the bed, and then reverse. He is drinking pretty well. Our volunteer is here in the morning while I go out. I tell Fred that he has to compromise with me and have someone here at least half the time and that I'm looking really bad. I left him alone, and he fell again on Saturday. They probably think I'm not taking good care of him. In his now strained voice, which is a higher sound and much weaker, he says, "You're doing a good job," and pats my arm. We make eye contact and smile at each other.

When I get home, the volunteer says he asked her when the nurse was coming to draw blood. He told her he was having it tested because he might be getting a transfusion.

Martha comes, and we go upstairs to check Fred's

vitals and draw blood. The right arm vein looks good, but looks are often deceiving, and she has to abandon that arm. The left arm yields right away, to her surprise and probably relief. We talk about when the results will be back and how a decision will be made on the transfusion. If he goes to the local hospital, Martha suggests that the hospice director temporarily act as Fred's doctor should something go wrong. I agree. When she leaves, I tell Fred the plan, and he nods and says again, "Thank you for asking for me." I suggest we move him before Kathy arrives if he still wants to go downstairs today. Yes, that probably makes sense. Thirty minutes before we start, I give him the 4 hour pain medication and an Ativan. I bring the oxygen a little closer, and it makes it almost to the bed. We get him up and around the bed to the walker. He rests, already gasping, while I fix the oxygen tube in place. Slowly, we walk toward the stairs. We get to the landing, and he has to sit down. Fortunately, there is a little stool there. Now he is four feet from the top of the stairs and sitting. He can't move. He's too weak to get himself up. He has the willpower, but he lacks the necessary strength. After some rest, I talk him into trying to move: "Let me lift you up, and we'll sit you on the top step." "How?" he says several times. I demonstrate how we will move and that I will hold him as he settles down on the stair. I pull him up when he's ready; he's getting so light, I think, and hold him to my body as I rotate him towards the top of the stair. He becomes nervous and wonders, "How will I get down?" I repeat, "You're going to sit down; just come down one step." It is his sheer will that is moving him. I try to gently let him down on the step while still holding on; he probably thinks he may fall down the stairs. Then we slide down one step at a time, resting in between. He is gasping for air, and after three steps, his head is hanging, and he says, "Lift my head." I hold his head up as we navigate a few more steps. Halfway down, he says, "Two at a time," overachieving to the end. We are almost at the bottom when Kathy arrives. As she enters the front door, I lean around the stairwell and tell her what we're doing. She asks, "Can I help?" I say, "We're OK," and she goes to the kitchen with dinner. Fred wants to get up before the bottom and swing around into the hospital bed. I encourage another step down, then I lift him up again, and we sidestep to the bottom of the bed. He falls onto the bed, and it takes some effort to get him situated—lifting his legs and pulling him up to the head of the bed. He cannot move. Finally, he is comfortable, and I head for the kitchen. I give Kathy a wide-eyed look with body language that says, "This is unbelievable." She gives me a big hug, and I cry a little. I talk about the day's struggle and the hope for a blood transfusion, with the expectation that it will perk him up. We talk for a while, and then I check on Fred. I have chilled champagne for us, and Kathy has it open when I return for fresh juice for Fred, who tells me the one by his bed is old. I chuckle at this; it's so typical that he wants everything to be very fresh. I'm glad his personality is still active. It takes Fred hours to recover from the move; the oxygen machine is on, but he's not sure it's helping. I give him a plate, and he takes a few bites. Kathy and I eat in the kitchen, and she asks how I am. I say, "It's getting harder; I'm worried that I have to move him and carry his weight and that my back will give out." She asks a few questions about our medical expenses and finances: are we living on our savings? Am I thinking about afterward?

I say, "I think about the future, but I have no specifics. I am focused on the vineyard; I can't lose the crop." She says, "No, you can't lose the crop. But what about you?" I say, "I don't know about me; I'll be 54 this year; I'm not young anymore. I think about security since I'll be alone." We agree that it's pretty safe here, and I have Tashie, dear Tashie. I give Fred his 12-hour and additional 4-hour pain medications to help him recover. After Kathy leaves, I gather blankets and two dog beds to sleep on in the living room. I assist Fred in using the commode before the lights go out. I have to lift him, and getting him back into bed is a struggle. He doesn't want to use the urinal; sitting on the commode is easier. The urination is slow. He gets up again in two hours, and we repeat the routine. The makeshift bed is so uncomfortable that Tashie has already abandoned it and gone upstairs to our bed. She's the smart one. My back is getting sore by the minute, and I finally tell Fred I can't lift him anymore, and I have to go upstairs to bed. At 4:30 a.m., he cries out, and I rush downstairs. He says he's been calling for a half hour. His voice is so weak, and he couldn't locate the bell I left for him to ring. He's slumped over, face-down on the mattress. I roll him over and slowly bring him up to a sitting position. I reposition the oxygen and wait while he rests. Again, I lift him from the bed and try to pivot him onto the commode, but each time it gets harder. Finally, I crawl back into bed for another hour of sleep.

Wednesday, March 3, 2004

The volunteer arrives around 9:30 a.m. I update her and start crying. I'm exhausted—physically and emotionally. She expresses sympathy and says, "I know you expected more time." Yes, there is never enough time. I tell her about the possible transfusion and that I expect phone calls this morning about the results. I tell her about the herculean effort to get him downstairs last night and that he is very unstable when he tries to stand. He'll probably not move until I get back.

When I return, there are several phone messages, one from the hospice nurse and one from Anne. It seems that the results were hemoglobin levels of 7.3. Last night, the hospice director and Dr. Cheng spoke and decided it was best for Fred to go back to Fox

Chase for the transfusion. They knew him best in case something happened. They also do some blood typing a little differently because of the chemotherapy drugs, which may make a difference. So, the messages say, "Get to Fox Chase by 10 a.m., and good luck." I pause to process this. Normally, it's good news; he should feel better, but the trip will not be easy. Since last Friday's trip for the abdominal drain, Fred's ability to move has significantly declined. I'm not sure he can walk to the car. I hope that he is recovering from the trip downstairs. Hoping at all may be false security. Last night was the worst night so far. I will prepare for the worst. Foreboding is pressing in on me.

I focus on liquids and small food portions. I offer to read, and he wants to rest. I wander to the kitchen area to do some work, and he calls out for me. This is the pattern for the afternoon. I have done no work for over a week. I bring the bills into the living room and think about moving another table into the living room so I can work standing up. The sitting plagues my back. Fred says he is so sorry I have to take care of him like this. I give him a big smile and say, "It's my pleasure. It's the least I can do; you have given me so many gifts." That is how I feel; I would gladly care for him like this to have him still with me. Last night's laxative is working, but the effort to get him up feels monumental. I leave the room for ten minutes and return to find Fred sprawled on the floor. I am pained to see him like this. I pick him up and maneuver his body to get him back into bed. It is not pretty, but I do my best not to hurt him. His legs seem a little stiff when I pick them up to swing them into bed. "Rough," he says. I say, "I'm sorry; I'm just trying to get you up quickly." Perhaps speed isn't required. Two hours later, he has to urinate, but it takes forever with little output. The evening repeats about every 2 hours when he is uncomfortable or has to go to the bathroom. He won't stay in bed to urinate. I say, "I have to sleep upstairs for my back. Please ring the bell." At 2 a.m., he cries out, and I find him again sprawled on the floor. I try to be a little gentler, but he is a total dead weight; he has no strength to help. It takes me at least thirty minutes to work him back into bed. I have lifted his weight at least five times for this one episode. I take a little extra muscle relaxer before going to bed. He cries for me again at 4:30 a.m. This time he is sitting on the bed. We have decided he doesn't need his clothes in bed; they're just a hassle to get off. He urinates and then lays back down but slips down from the top of the bed again. He has to have his upper body raised because of the surgical reconfiguration. "Lift me," he says again. I try to half-lift and half-pull him up. It's a little better. I check the clock; it's 5 a.m., and I set the alarm for 6:30 a.m.

Thursday, March 4, 2004

He's finally resting when I come downstairs. I take my coffee and think about how to make today work. The result is for him to have more energy, which is worth the effort, but I don't know about tomorrow and the abdominal drain. I'll take it one day at a time.

I check the wheelchair and take it to the front door. This will be its first use. Fred is awake and asks what time we will leave. I say, "Around 8:30 a.m. Do you have to go to the bathroom?" "No," he says, nodding but not moving. I ask, "Would you like some breakfast?" "No," he says, nodding. I say, "OK, I'll get your pills." It takes some time to take them. Each pill takes about one minute.

I call Barbara and Jon and ask them to come over and help me get Fred into the car. Yes, they will be over. They have experience moving their parents in wheelchairs. Their assistance—and primarily their assistance— gets Fred up and into the wheelchair and out the door, down a few steps, down the walk, and finally into the car. As they are getting him situated in the wheelchair, I am talking to Tashie, telling her where we're going and how long we will be gone. Fred calls out for me to stop talking to the dog! We all glance at each other, and I approach Fred and hold his hand. Jon has moved the oxygen machine by the front door. They put the portable oxygen tank in the car. I think it is for 4 hours. We get it set up and on Fred before setting out. Down the hill, Fred remembers his red card, which is always in his wallet. Going back is the better option. Tashie is now used to us coming back for something we forgot. She is nonplussed to see me, and I don't engage in further conversation.

Fred nods on the trip. I have brought the medications, a urinal, and our book. I know we can get help when we get there, but we should have our wheelchair, which is too small, in the back just in case theirs' are already in use. I pull up in front and wait for the volunteer. As he gets the chair, I take Fred's red card and the prescriptions into the lab area to check him in. I have to leave him by the front door while I go park the car. Then we go into the lab/infusion room waiting area. I have all the other stuff in a big bag that keeps falling off my shoulder. I leave the oxygen in the car, hoping they have some there. I notice the bigger tanks on wheels and remember we have those also; that's what I should have brought. I hope they take us soon. Shortly, a nurse comes to take us in for the blood draw. They will access his port for the transfusion. She flushes the other side and treats him oh so nicely. Thank God for Fox Chase, the embarrassment at the county hospital was beyond my patience. It's too noisy in the waiting room, so we go to another quiet sitting area. I get him some juice and tea for myself. I give him extra Ativan and pain medications. I am reading the grape spray manual and asking a few questions, but mostly trying to hold his hand. He is wearing his new Cape Cod hat and trying to hide his face. In less than an hour, the infusion room nurse calls for him. I wave, gather our things, and push his chair towards that door. I notice the supervisor nurse come out through the door. We don't make eye contact after the incident where she practically yelled at me last fall. She turns around, opens the door, and holds it for us with her eyes turned down. Fred waves as we go through the doorway. It feels like everyone is looking at us as I wheel him to his chair. We are now the patient worse than the others, in a lot of pain, and on our last hope. Another nurse helps get Fred into his chair. Our nurse starts talking to me.

"Are you the only family here?" I reply, "Yes."

"Is he off hospice?" I reply, "Not as far as I know."

I ask how long it will take for the transfusion. My mother will be visiting, and I am thinking of going out.

"Your father will be here for at least 4 hours." It's 11:30 a.m.

I say, "He's my husband." Poor Fred, he really hates this part. This pauses the nurse as she looks at Fred and back at me. And I tell her it really bothers him. She says, "He can probably hear us." I nod. I am busy trying to make him a little more comfortable; it's probably impossible, but I try. They hook him up for pre-medications, Tylenol, and antihistamines right away. I sit and wait, trying not to look at anyone else, for they are looking at me.

The nurse returns and asks Fred if he wants to be resuscitated, which causes me to panic. She says, "This is really a formality; nothing will happen to him." I say, "Yes, resuscitate him and call Dr. Cheng." Then I tell her about the medications I have brought and the urinal. She thanks me, and I leave them on the small tabletop. She asks about oxygen. I say I have only a small portable tank in the car. She says no problem; they have everything there, and she attaches a hose to the outlet and sets the rate. I say that "2" doesn't seem like enough; she will try "3," and I watch as she hooks the hose around Fred's ears and under the chin—a new way to put the hose on. Maybe this is more comfortable. I make a mental note. I try to read as I wait for Mom to arrive. She enters the room at 12:30 p.m. Fred doesn't look up as I greet her. His head is hanging down. I kiss him and say, "I am going out for awhile." He looks at me with alarm, and the nurse comes over and says, "He will be fine; he'll probably be sleeping for the whole time." Mom says hello to Fred, he waves, and we depart, weaving through the infusion room full of patients and family.

We grab a quick lunch, and then I leave for the local Y, feeling a little guilty but knowing I need to take care of myself. No one knows me there; there are no questions to answer. I call Jon and Barbara to give an update, then return a few calls. The solar grants have been verbally approved, and we're ready to order the equipment. Will Fred be here to see it? The path looks very perilous.

I arrive back in the infusion room at three. The second unit will take about 45 minutes longer. He's awake and waiting quietly. The urinal is empty, and the medications are untouched. Yes, that's how he would handle the day—no food or water. But now he has to urinate. I tell his nurse, and we draw the curtains. The nurse tries to help hold the urinal. After 5 minutes, she says maybe she should leave and mouths to me, "To give him privacy." I nod and continue to hold the urinal. This is the routine now: 5–10 minutes before he can urinate. After he finishes, I look around to dispose of the liquid; the bathroom is in use. I ask the nurse for a wheelchair, and she asks, "Are you taking care of him alone?" "Yes." I say, nodding, and she looks at me for a minute. I say, "It's getting difficult of late. He's fallen, and I have to pick him up; I've been struggling." She simply shakes her head and walks away, leaving me to lift Fred out of the infusion chair and into the wheelchair, another lift on my own. We make it, I get my things, and slowly we make our way out of the infusion room. Someone holds the door. My gaze is fixed ahead; I avoid eye contact and stand tall. My eyes well up with tears; I hope Fred doesn't see. I figure out that the upper drop-off inside the garage is the way to go. I tell Fred, and he says, "Yes, I thought that too." We enter the car and take off by 4 p.m., just before rush-hour traffic. I call Barbara and Jon and tell them we should be home by 5:30 p.m. I check on Fred frequently to see if he is more lively. He says there is no difference. We arrive before our friends. I get the door open and the oxygen going, and then they are here, may God bless them ,fully taking over and moving him into the too-small wheelchair and then into the house. I noticed that going out of the house, the back of the wheelchair was breaking the door threshold—more stuff to fix, so I suggest we go in feet first, which worked. They get him back into bed and move the oxygen machine into the next room; it sounds like a small generator. I get him some fresh Gatorade, hoping to replace the electrolytes and more pain medications. He nods off to sleep, and our friends bring fresh bread, soup, and eggs for supper. I open our champagne and relax for a moment. They bring in the big box on the porch—the new air mattress I ordered from LL Bean—so I can sleep in the living room with Fred. When I open it, it's not an air mattress; it's a hamper! It's unbelievable. You have to double-check everything in this country. Productivity may be up, but carelessness and mistakes are higher than ever. I call Bean; they are slightly surprised, but not too much, and will get something out tomorrow. But no carrier delivers to our area on Saturdays. We're only one hour from Philadelphia, but you would think we're in Alaska. Finally, I have them send it to my sister's in Reading for Saturday delivery. Our friends have a foam mattress they will bring over later. I keep checking on Fred, fearful of some reaction to the transfusion. I open the envelope my 6-year-old nephew left for Fred on Tuesday. He wrote to Uncle Fred that he hoped he wouldn't die. This chokes me up. Fred looks at me with big eyes. I squeeze his hand and leave the room. He is resting now, and I clear a path on the dining room table, and we sit and enjoy a repast together. For a brief moment, I feel normal again. Fred is still resting, so I go to the video store while they stand guard. They bring up the apnea. "I know," I say, and the hospice literature talks about that as a symptom of dying. They look at me. I know what they are thinking, but I will not go down that path. They leave as we start to get absorbed by Survivor, one of the few activities that Fred can stay with. An hour later, I leave the room and return to find Fred again on the floor. It dismays me; I feel helpless and know he must be hurting. "Pick me up," he says again as I muster the strength. I get him settled back in bed and try to pull him up. We work the bed to help his position. It is not the best, but it will have to do. He is quiet for the rest of the evening. I fall comfortably asleep on the floor of the room. Tashie tries to take over the middle of the foam mattress, and Larry, our cat, perches near my head and chews on my hair—a weird thing he likes to do. Three times during the night, Fred wakes me—he is sitting up and wants to go on the commode. We have this "not-really-well-worked-out" routine where I lift him, and he pauses mid-air as I pull down the sweats and undies and then lower him onto the commode. It's not working tonight, and it takes several tries and long waits in between as he catches his breath. One time he stands straight up on his own, and I say that must be the transfusion—maybe it's finally helping. We stay standing, his arm around my shoulder; he is still strong, and for a moment, I pretend that nothing is wrong, and we share a hug. I tell him, "Tomorrow, you'll be stronger. Jen will be here on Saturday."

Friday, March 5, 2004

He sleeps in a little. He's very tired from yesterday. I wake him to give him his morning medications. Each pill is harder to swallow. He can't take them all at once. He sleeps until late morning while I do paperwork. When he wakes, I ask about food. He's not hungry. I remind him that if he is going to see the new shoots, he will have to eat. He eventually agrees to cereal. We talk about our will. I say I have called the lawyer our friend recommended. We discuss a few changes, and I explain that we need separate wills. It is mostly a formality now, but I want to know his wishes. He will think about it. I go out after lunch to the Y and get groceries. Kathy will come over tonight. I have everyone come to the kitchen door to minimize disruption for Fred. I cook a pork roast with roasted vegetables. Kathy and I drink champagne as I prepare Fred's plate. She says, "Aren't you going to cut that up?" It had never occurred to me. That would mean Fred couldn't do it. I cut up the meat and put a little more gravy on it. I sit with him a little while he eats, keeping my plate in the kitchen. He says it tastes good, and he eats a lot of it. I think of all the recent meals and that it has probably been hard for him to cut the meat—so stupid of me. He asks when Kathy will leave, wanting us to be alone. We sit for the evening mostly in silence. He wants to stay up late and nap frequently. Just when I turn the lights out, he sits up. He tries to urinate for a long while. Then we try to get him on the commode. It is not pretty, and he is holding onto the bed and wants me to hold his head up. As he tries to stand up and I try to lift him, he slumps to the floor. I am afraid he has banged his back. I struggle to lift him and finally get him to the kneeling position. Then, with great effort, we get him onto the bed, but he is lying face down. "Pick me up," is all he can say. This is not dignified, and I am horrified that I can't do better. Finally, I brace my right leg folded onto the bed and use the side of my body to roll and lift him over. I say, "Hold onto the rail as I move you." "What's happening to me?" he says. I say, "You're weak from the transfusion." I get him some fresh juice with ice and more medications. I lay down, feeling exhausted. He calms down in about 30 minutes. And we both get some rest. At 4 a.m., he is sitting up again, and we repeat the whole agonizing effort to urinate again. Up and down on the bed, leaning over, trying and failing to sit on the commode. Gasping, he flops back in bed, and again we struggle to get him up to the top, his feet hanging over, a sip of juice, and more medications; he seems anxious or restless. Finally, his breathing calms down. I flop on the floor mattress; my eyes closed, before I pull the covers up.

Saturday, March 6, 2004

Dawn is breaking as my eyes open. They look at Fred first, and he is looking at me with very big, soft blueish eyes. I am startled; his eyes are touching my soul. I ask, "What? Are you alright?" He nods, "Yes." We hold each other's eyes for a moment. He is now looking through me. "I'm here," I say. I feel very tired and close my eyes. I must have fallen right back asleep. The next thing I know, he says, "Janet," as loud as he can. His voice changed several months ago and is getting weaker. I bolt upright. "What?" I blurt out; he is looking at me. "Do you have to go?" I ask "Yes."

I clamber up from the floor, thankful for several hours' sleep. We go to work, trying to help him get up and onto the commode. He has to sit down several times. We try the urinal in various positions; most of them are unsuccessful. In the end, he and the bed are all wet. He says to leave it. Classic Fred: nothing is too uncomfortable. I say, "No, that's not good." And we work on rolling him over to one side to put dry towels under him. I check his clothes, change everything, and leave the bottom half naked. He reluctantly agrees, asking if the nurse is coming today. I get him his medications and fresh juice. He asks, "What day is this?" I reply, "Saturday; Jen will be here tonight. Are you comfortable?"

He says, "No."

We struggle together to get him pulled up. I make him promise not to get up. I say, "I'm going to have to put the sides up on the bed if you keep trying to get up." We look at each other, and I melt thinking about how totally dehumanizing this is for Fred. I say, "What can I do to make it more comfortable?"

He says, "Nothing."

"Would you like me to read our book?" I say, grabbing a chair, and I sit close.

"Later," he says, sighing and closes his eyes.

I sit for a while, then think about my schedule for the day. I call our friends again to come over while I go out. When I tell Fred, he says, "Don't stay gone too long." Two hours, our agreed-to absence time.

I call on the way home to say I'll be there soon. Of course, he hasn't moved since I left. I ask our friends to stay while the lawyer comes. Jon read the draft to Fred while I was gone. The lawyer arrives at 11, and we spend a little while discussing the document and changes Fred, and I have decided on. I walk the lawyer out and quickly show him the winery. He inquires about Fred's prognosis and is taken aback by the short time frame. They had a nice conversation.

As soon as our friends leave, he pushes the covers over and tries to get up. "No," I say, "Let me help you." We somehow manage to get him onto the commode, but he can't go. I can't pull him or lift him. My strength is not there. He falls forward onto the bed. I push him backward, and he flops on the floor. This is terrible. He is in a heap on the floor, unable to move, and I am in a panic, trying to think of how to get him up. I hear a delivery truck and look out to find that Medical Home Products is here to exchange the wheelchair. I leave Fred momentarily, go to the door, and explain that my husband is using the commode; please wait outside. After another struggle to lift him, I get him up to his knees again. I push his middle onto the bed, hoping I am not hurting him too much. I brace my leg against him and pull his legs up. It isn't pretty, but he is at least off the floor. Actually, this is pathetic, and I think, "This shouldn't be like this." I can't continue to help him alone. I can't move him around—he is still a big man. I tell Fred I will ask the Medical Home Products guy to help me move him. "But I don't have anything on," he says. I say, "I'll keep you covered; he will be understanding." I go to the door and start crying that I need help to move my husband; would he please help? He moves instantly toward the door, and I say loud enough for Fred to hear that my husband does not have underwear on, and I have him partially covered. He nods and looks at Fred, mercifully showing no reaction to what must look like poor care on my part. He is strong and talks to Fred about lifting him. He gently picks Fred up and repositions him on the bed. He asks Fred if that is comfortable and adjusts his body position again. Fred says, "Yes, that's good." I am so relieved. We talk about other equipment to help move Fred, like a kind of lift, and I ask for a bed table like in the hospital. "Yes, we have those." Why don't we already have one? He says, "I can bring these by later that day if the nurse orders them."

I say, "Thank you; God bless you."

I tell Fred, "I'm sorry, but I don't think I can move him anymore; my back is sore, and we will be a sorry couple if I am unable to move." I calm down and get him something fresh to drink, more medications, and my lunch. I sit with him until the nurse comes. He's too tired for me to read. When Martha arrives, I update her on our conversation from yesterday. I tell her I can't do this alone. She talks about my hiring a live-in nurse. How much is that? I think about how I might manage that. She comes prepared to help clean Fred and calmly shows me how to do that, gently moving him from side to side. She inspects the marks and bruises on his back from the falls. She dresses one and then cleans his back with a special cleaning spray and lotion. I clean his genital area and then cover him up. Then I get his toothbrush, dental floss, and mouthwash for him to work on his teeth with a spit bowl. I have clean clothes ready, but she suggests we cut the tops in the back, so we dress him from the front. I say, "Really?" I rethink the clothing and come back with older shirts. She also shows me how to roll him from side to side, changing the bed. We put clean sheets on and then a plastic trash bag with another sheet on top for easy changing. Fred seems relaxed, and I know he appreciates the gentle, calm handling. Martha suggests a personal aid, and that could be every day. I say yes to that, thinking a man can help me move him more easily. We discuss the medications; they don't seem to work well. I am thinking of doubling the long-acting pain medication, and she also says that's what she thinks. We go over what is the maximum we can be using. Fred is tired and quiet when she leaves. She comments that he seems comfortable. I say, "That's only while you're here. As soon as you leave, he'll want to get up and start moving." "Oh?" she says.

I lay down on the floor, and we both have a little rest. I awake after sundown, and the house is dark and a little chilly. I turn up the heat and check on Fred. He opens his eyes, and I give him a smile and a soft kiss. I say, "I'm sorry it's been so rough over the last day; I'll try harder." He squeezes my hand and says, "You're doing a good job." I get the pain relievers and fresh soda and suggest some dinner options. A repeat of last night is the only choice. He eats a little, and we search for something on the 600 channels of Direct TV. I find a history show and fall asleep in the chair. At 9 p.m., Fred asks when Jennifer will arrive; I check the time and estimate she will arrive around 11 p.m. He doesn't need to use the commode and lays quietly in bed. I flop on the floor and rest for a moment. The noise in the driveway turns out to be the Medical Products truck bringing the hoist and hospital table. We settle down again with all the lights on. The next thing I know, Jen is pulling into the driveway. "Jen's here," I say as I get up. Fred's eyes are open, and looking out the window. I greet her at the door, and she greets Fred with a big smile. I know he has greatly declined since she last saw him—only four weeks ago—but she doesn't react with alarm. They talk for a moment. I go to the kitchen to close up for the night, and Jen follows me. She asks, "Is my Dad OK?" I say, "Well, he has declined since you saw him." That is enough for tonight. We all decide to go to bed, and Jen says not to let her sleep in too late. I promise and hug her.

At 2 a.m., Fred sits up, trying to get my attention. I am much more tired than I was ten days ago when I would awake at the slightest movement. We try to get him on the commode and can't make it. He then decides he has to urinate. We try multiple positions, and nothing comes out. After a half hour, he wants to get on the commode again. He tries to get up with me lifting him but falls back on the bed. "Pick me up," he says, and I pull him up to sit. I pull the walker over for him to hold onto as I try to position the commode closer. We try many maneuvers without success. Each time I try to lift or pull, his body feels like dead weight. We've been at this for hours. Suddenly his body relaxes, and the bowels move. As this happens, he flops across the bed, and I fear he has hit his head. His head is arched back, his eyes are very big, and his breathing has stopped. I think, "No! Not like this," and simultaneously realize that is what will happen when he dies—he will stop breathing. "Breathe, Fred, breathe!" I say loudly and push his chest. I say it again, and he jerks and gasps again. "What's happening?" he says almost immediately. I say, "It's probably the laxative from yesterday working its way through your system. Maybe that wasn't a good idea." I tell him to stay still while I get some things to clean him up. I say, "It's alright, don't worry; I just have to get a few towels." I try to be calm and work quickly but gently. I think about waking Jen, but decide this is not a dignified view of her father. I roll him over and clean him up with the new spray cleaners. This works well, and shortly I am ready to pull out the sheet. I roll him from side to side and get a fresh towel under him—the best I can do. "What's happening?" he says again. "It's OK, it was just an accident; everything is fine." I say this as I sort out the possibilities in my mind. "Don't go away," he says.

I say, "I won't, I'm right here, I'm going to lie down again, call me if you need anything."

Bad night.

Sunday, March 7, 2004

7 a.m.: He continues to want to try to get up. I try to reposition him. I say, "Is that better?"

He says, "No," and glares at me.

I give him two four-hour medications. He's restless, trying to get out of bed. I say, "No, you have to stay there."

He says, "I have to get up."

I ask, "Where are you going?"

"To find out what's going on with me," he says with perfect authority. In any other situation, this would sound normal. I try to sooth him and pick his legs up, telling him to lie down. He grimaces when I move his legs. His feet seem a little more swollen and cold.

"Stay with me," he says.

I say, "I'm not going anywhere."

He says, "Hold me."

I sit and hold his hand and stroke his face.

He says, "Talk to me." I can't remember him ever saying this before.

I say, "OK, do you just want me to chatter away? Or something specific?"

No response.

I say, "About what's happening to you?"

He gives a nod and a grimace.

I ask, "Are you in pain?" Another nod.

I say, "Wait for a minute, I will get something."

"Don't go far," he says, maintaining eye contact with me.

"I won't," I say and dash to the dining room to grab the 12-hour medications. I rush back and say, "One more minute—I will get fresh juice." I give him the pills. It's getting more difficult for him to take them. I wait minutes between each pill. He'll never be able to take the regular AM pills. Yesterday either. We sit, and I hold his hand, periodically kiss him, and rub his head where the baby hairs are coming in. He vacillates between being anxious and exhausted. He tries to get up again, and I gently push him back. I ask, "Do you have to go to the bathroom again?"

He says, "No."

We sit quietly again. I gently stroke his hand and face and say, "Best buddy," and he whispers back, "Best buddy."

8 a.m.: "What's happening to me?" he asks again. After a moment, I look into his eyes, pause, and say with empathy and great sadness, "You're dying." It is the first time I have ever said these words.

"Who says?" he quickly replies with strength—a quick challenge response—his signature.

I say, "Well, your nurse and your doctor."

He asks, "Am I dead?"

I reply, "No."

He asks, "When will I die?"

I reply, "They don't know when." My brain engages for a moment, and I recall bits of the stories in the book "Final Gifts."

Then I ask, "Do you know when?"

He says, "Today, I will die today."

He looks at me with wide eyes that are bluer.

He says it matter-of-factly.

It's surreal; we're two souls holding hands, with only love and knowledge passing between us. The world does not exist. I think I can feel the circle of angels around us. I say, "Wait, don't move," and rush to the back stairs and call up for Jen to get up. I return to Fred's bed and say, "Jen is getting up." He looks at me and through me at the same time. That is the look I saw yesterday morning when I awoke at dawn to find him looking at me with those very big eyes. I hear Jen in the kitchen and again say, "Wait, I'll be right back."

"Hurry back," he says.

In the kitchen, I give Jen a moment and ask, "Did you sleep well?" Then I say, "Come to see your father." She pulls up the chair on the other side of the bed, and I repeat the conversation Fred and I just had. She looks at her father with wide eyes, holding his hand, with tears streaming down her face. She looks at me as if to say, "Really?" We sit and hold his hands and give him kisses. She tells him how much she loves him and assures him that everything will be fine, Olivia loves Grandpa Fred, and she will show Olivia all the wonderful and important things he showed her, and she will miss him very much.

I squeeze his hand, and he squeezes back. He's still here. I stroke his head and ask him if he's comfortable. He shakes his head, "No." "My poor best buddy," I say, and he answers back, "Best buddy." I get a round of medications and some fresh juice as Jen sits with him. "Is that helping yet?" I ask after about thirty minutes. He gives another head shake and says, "No." He grimaces. I give him another pain pill and an Ativan. I stroke his hand, and he says, "Rough," and pulls his hand back. I say, "Sorry," and try not to touch him with my fingertips, which feel like sandpaper from the frostbite. It's a very small way for him to be in charge. There's been so little over the last 20 months that he can control.

"Help me," he says. I ask, "Are you in pain?" He gives a nod and a grimace. I look at Jen—what to do?—the emergency kit. I go and grab it from the bottom of the refrigerator. I get the folder and check which drug is for pain. It's the liquid—a very small amount in the bottom and a short eye dropper. I'm able to draw up the correct amount, ½ cc.

I ask Fred to open his mouth and lift his tongue, and I dispense the liquid. Then I call the hospice number and ask for Martha to be paged. They ask what is wrong, and I say, "My husband just told me that he will die today." She responds quickly and says to wait a moment as she will try to get someone on the phone now. No one is there on Sunday morning, but Martha will get the page.

"How are you now? Any relief?" I ask Fred. He says, "No." I look at Jen. What else can we do? The phone rings, and as I pull away, Fred says, "Don't go far." I kiss him and say, "I'm only going to answer the phone; I'm here, my best buddy." Martha wants to know what has happened. I tell the story since she was here yesterday. As I talk, I ask, "Is it possible that Fred thought I was saying when he might die? That I had put the thought in his head?" I ask Martha, and she says that's what she thinks because his vital signs were all good yesterday. She wouldn't have thought he would die today. And then I say, "But the stories in the book are all about the patient knowing when they will die." She says, "Yes, you are doing all the right things. Give him the liquid pain medication every two hours." She can't get here till around 3 p.m., as planned. I call Barbara and Jon, tell them the story, and ask that they come over. "Yes," they always say yes. It is still amazing to me that those who have surrounded us respond to my requests with gracious unselfishness.

Fred remains anxious and in pain. Jen and I sit with him and try to comfort him. His breathing is about the same—apneic long moments that feel like 5 minutes but are only 20 seconds. I continue to say, "Breathe, Fred, breathe," and he does. Jon and Barbara come over and stay in the room. At one point, they are talking, and Fred opens his eyes and motions with his hands to ask for quiet. The minutes tick by, and our attempts to comfort him do not ease his pain. Periodically his breathing pauses are too long for me, and I say again, "Breathe, Fred, breathe," and he does. And often, I will squeeze his hand, kiss his head, and say, "Best buddy," and he immediately responds in a soft voice, "Best buddy," and we squeeze our hands together again. Two hours go by, and I give the next dose of liquid morphine. Thankfully, he starts to relax and falls asleep. At 11:30 a.m., Jen and I go to the kitchen to see about food, and our friends leave. I start watering the orchids and call Kathy. I tell her about Fred's earlier conversation. She is quiet for a moment and says, "Really?" We talk about the conversation with the nurse and how I might have suggested that he was dying today. But the patients know, so we are waiting for the nurse now, and he is finally resting. She says not to leave him, to stay with him. "Do you mean don't be in the kitchen watering plants?" I say facetiously. She says, "Do you want me to come down?" "Yes," I say with tears. She calls Mom, who leaves immediately to come here.

Then I remember the lawyer. He will make the changes and bring them back to sign on Monday. Should I call him? I decide to wait a little longer. The minutes tick by, and Fred is still resting. His breathing is more relaxed, although apnea is still happening. He always responds to, "Breathe, Fred, breathe." At 1:00 p.m., I decide to call the lawyer. I tell him Fred has taken a turn for the worse and ask, "Can they get here as early as possible tomorrow? After a pause I say "Can you come as soon as possible?" He thinks momentarily and says, "I will call you back within 15 minutes," and we hang up. I continue to sit with Fred. The phone rings five minutes later, and the lawyer says, "We'll be there in one hour." At 1:30 p.m., Fred is still relaxed and sleeping. I talk to Jen about the lawyer coming and Fred signing the papers. We discuss how that will happen and conclude that I must help him. But he's due for the liquid morphine at 1:30 p.m.; should I give it to him now or wait a little? I don't know if I can wake him up. I am torn about what to do. I don't want him to be in pain. Jen and I decide to wait a while. At 2:30 p.m., Fred is alert and anxious. His legs hurt. He cries out for help. I run for the liquid morphine. We try to comfort him. The lawyer arrives with two witnesses. Jen and I have the hospital table tilted for writing. We decide it's OK for me to help Fred sign the papers. He waves at the visitors in acknowledgment. The lawyer repeats the will changes for him, and he says it doesn't matter. I help him hold the pen while he signs the documents. "Please wait a moment because Fred has a special book for his granddaughter that he wants to sign," I say, and I simply sign the book "To Olivia from Grandpa Fred," foregoing the idea of a more meaningful message. The visitors comment on how that is the most important thing—a message for a granddaughter—and everyone smiles. I have Jen walk them out and show them the winery, and give them each a bottle of wine. Once they leave, Fred is again crying out for help. He's in pain, and his legs are hurting. Mom and I try to reposition his legs, which are more swollen and stiffer. Martha arrives just then. She quickly assesses Fred and asks what has happened since we talked. We review the medication amounts and frequencies. She says we can double the frequency and start doing that. Earlier in the morning, she had arranged for a new prescription, and Jon and Barbara had driven the half hour each way to pick it up. We start giving him a dose every 30 minutes. Nothing is happening. He complains about his leg—it hurts, and nothing we do is helping. Martha is in the kitchen talking with the doctors, following their escalation process. She comes back and says we must try to comfort him and give it some time; she will be getting a call back from the Fox Chase doctor. There is no comforting him. Jen and I hold his hands and try to reposition him. I say, "Best buddy," we're trying to help. "Best buddy," he replies in a whisper and rests momentarily. Then it starts again, and he cries out for help. After an hour of this, I go to the kitchen doorway and say loudly to Martha, who is on the phone, "Can't you do something? He is crying out in pain!" I return to Fred, racking my brain for something that would help. He thrashes, grimaces, and cries, "Help me," and has brief quiet moments. Little pieces of my heart are torn away with each "Help me." His breathing is getting more labored; his chest is heaving. Martha increases the liquid morphine, giving him doses every fifteen minutes, and says someone is coming with a morphine drip.

After two hours, he starts to calm down, but his breathing is very labored. I lean close to his head, say, "Best buddy," and rest my cheek on his. There is no reply. It's 6:00 p.m. I sit and hold his hand while people come and go. Bonnie and Doug come by and sit in the room for a while, looking at Fred. Bonnie then walks over to Fred, leans down as if kissing him, and whispers something in his ear with an air of intimacy. I am stunned and perplexed by her actions, and she turns to say, "I told him now he will believe in God!" I'll save my agitated feelings for another day.

The hospice morphine drip crew arrives at about 7:30 p.m. I now know there will be no return. He will die today. More papers to sign, a controlled substance. They talk among themselves, and then the emergency nurse starts to talk to me: "Have you made your peace?" "Yes," I say. She asks the same of Jennifer. "Yes," she says. His vitals are slowing down; his heart rate is so slow that they believe he will go when they start the drip. So, it all comes down to this. I remember when he asked me some weeks back, in an anguished moment, "What do I think about at the end?" I was helpless then, and I feel helpless now. He seems peaceful, and Jen and I tell him again that we love him. There is nothing more for me to say.

The house is full of lit candles, creating a soft atmosphere through the early evening. The hospice crew needs full lighting. I watch with slight academic interest as they access his port. The light feels harsh, and the room now feels sterile. Jen and I are still holding his hands, which feel limp, as they start the pump. They are all watching the patient, my husband, Fred. In a moment, he takes his last breath.

After a minute or so, one of the nurses walks to the kitchen; I assume to tell my family. Later, I discover that the hospice workers went to the kitchen to dispose of the narcotic prescriptions. A family member asked and was then told that Fred had passed away. The next thirty minutes are a blur of telephone calls from the funeral home and communications for the hospice group. I sit and hold Fred's hand while they surround me with the various papers and messages. I half listen, as I am still with Fred. The funeral director wants to come out immediately to get the body. I say, "No, he will stay here." Then he explains that the law allows for 24 hours for cremation. He agrees to pick Fred up in the morning but cautions me with stories of the body doing strange things. The hospice folk are all smiling; it was a successful death for them. The disparities in viewpoints are strange. I want my husband back; there is nothing successful for me here. I feel empty when I go to bed. I decide not to sleep in the living room with Fred. Mom sleeps over in my room on the borrowed foam mattress. In the middle of the night, I go downstairs for another moment with Fred. The stars are shining brightly.

Will to Live: 0

Cancer: 1

Afterword

Life Goes On

It's hard to think about anything besides your personal war. Your own life and the patient's are seemingly suspended, but the forces of life do not stop. Life continues around you.

We are "glorified farmers" because we grow wine grapes, but farmers are reliant on and linked to nature's cycle.

The diagnosis occurred in that brief late-season pause before the crush of harvest. Harvesting at a winery means constant overload. The gods may have picked this time for us because we would be driven by the necessary activity of the "crush." It gave me a break from the constant, overwhelming, deafening roar that is life-threatening cancer.

People who don't know about your situation act as they always have, unaware that you are crippled inside, always on the verge of tears, and wishing that someone would please just make it right.

So you pretend, a smile plastered on your face, chin up, and be positive, belying your true feelings and the total terror you wake up with every day. Your world is changed, and you are in a cycle of ever-changing information about the patient. And just when you think it's getting stable, something will crash down on you repeatedly. Until you finally give up the pretense that you have any control over the situation. You are only along for the ride.

The circle of people who know your situation behaves in a new way. They are supportive and sympathetic and respect your space. The problem is that life just doesn't stop. If only you could be spared more pain, but that is not the case.

Life is teaching me more lessons, but I don't want any more.

Now I almost hate to ask people how they are; maybe that's why some people don't ask.

Drugs

Besides the chemotherapy drugs, the patient may need any or all of the following:

Anti-anxiety drugs.

Anti-depressants.

Anti-nausea drugs.

Appetite stimulators, e.g., steroids.

Anti-acid drugs.

Anti-diarrhea drugs.

Anti-constipation drugs.

Antibiotics.

Heart medications.

And the need may last a long time. I am not a proponent of drugs, but I know for a fact, that cancer patients are in a separate class of need. They need all the help available on this planet.

Chemotherapy

Its purpose is to kill your immune system and all the live cells it comes in contact with.

Radiation

Its purpose is to dematerialize the cancer mass.

Meanwhile, the Patient is...

Fighting the war,

afraid to face the light of day,

reeling with disbelief and shocked beyond belief,

terrified of the dark and of what comes next,

steeling himself for the fight,

unable to move, think, care,

alone, beyond connection,

viewing from a lonely island,

that he alone knows.

www.ingramcontent.com/pod-product-compliance
Lightning Source LLC
Chambersburg PA
CBHW020048170426
43199CB00009B/214